Rehabilitation from the Perspective of the Athletic Trainer/Physical Trainer

Guest Editor

JEFF G. KONIN, PhD, ATC, PT

CLINICS IN SPORTS MEDICINE

www.sportsmed.theclinics.com

Consulting Editor
MARK D. MILLER, MD

January 2010 • Volume 29 • Number 1

SAUNDERS an imprint of ELSEVIER, Inc.

W.B. SAUNDERS COMPANY
A Division of Elsevier Inc.

1600 John F. Kennedy Blvd. • Suite 1800 • Philadelphia, Pennsylvania 19103

http://www.theclinics.com

CLINICS IN SPORTS MEDICINE Volume 29, Number 1
January 2010 ISSN 0278-5919, ISBN-13: 978-1-4377-1873-7

Editor: Ruth Malwitz
Developmental Editor: Donald Mumford

Clinics in Sports Medicine (ISSN 0278-5919) is published quarterly by Elsevier Inc., 360 Park Avenue South, New York, NY 10010-1710. Months of issue are January, April, July, and October. Business and Editorial Offices: 1600 John F. Kennedy Blvd., Ste. 1800, Philadelphia, PA 19103-2899. Customer Service Office: 3251 Riverport Lane, Maryland Heights, MO 63043. Periodicals postage paid at New York, NY and additional mailing offices. Subscription prices are $278.00 per year (US individuals), $424.00 per year (US institutions), $140.00 per year (US students), $315.00 per year (Canadian individuals), $512.00 per year (Canadian institutions), $195.00 (Canadian students), $382.00 per year (foreign individuals), $512.00 per year (foreign institutions), and $195.00 per year (foreign students). Foreign air speed delivery is included in all *Clinics* subscription prices. All prices are subject to change without notice. **POSTMASTER:** Send address changes to *Clinics in Sports Medicine*, Elsevier Health Sciences Division, Subscription Customer Service, 3251 Riverport Lane, Maryland Heights, MO 63043. Customer Service (orders, claims, online, change of address): Elsevier Health Sciences Division, Subscription Customer Service, 3251 Riverport Lane, Maryland Heights, MO 63043. Tel: 1-800-654-2452 (U.S. and Canada); 314-447-8871 (outside U.S. and Canada). Fax: 314-447-8029. E-mail: journalscustomerservice-usa@elsevier.com (for print support); journalsonlinesupport-usa@elsevier.com (for online support).

Reprints. For copies of 100 or more of articles in this publication, please contact the Commercial Reprints Department, Elsevier Inc., 360 Park Avenue South, New York, NY 10010-1710. Tel.: 212-633-3812; Fax: 212-462-1935; E-mail: reprints@elsevier.com.

Clinics in Sports Medicine is covered in *MEDLINE/PubMed (Index Medicus) Current Contents/Clinical Medicine, Excerpta Medica,* and *ISI/Biomed.*

Printed and bound by CPI Group (UK) Ltd, Croydon, CR0 4YY

Transferred to Digital Print 2011

Contributors

CONSULTING EDITOR

MARK D. MILLER, MD
S. Ward Casscells Professor of Orthopaedic Surgery, University of Virginia, Charlottesville, Virginia; Team Physician, James Madison University, Harrisonburg, Virginia

GUEST EDITOR

JEFF G. KONIN, PhD, ATC, PT
Associate Professor and Vice Chair, Department of Orthopaedics and Sports Medicine; Executive Director, Sports Medicine and Athletic Related Trauma (SMART) Institute, University of South Florida, Tampa, Florida

AUTHORS

BRAIN ARMSTRONG, MPT
Physical Therapist, Methodist Sports Medicine Center/The Orthopaedic Specialists, Indianapolis, Indiana

CHAD ASPLUND, MD
Clinical Assistant Professor, Department of Family Medicine, Division of Sports Medicine, The Ohio State University, Columbus, Ohio

JENNIFER BROWN, ATC
Associate Athletic Trainer, Northwestern University Department of Intercollegiate Sports Medicine, Evanston, Illinois

MARK DE CARLO, PT, DPT, MHA, SCS, ATC
Vice President Clinical Operations, Physical Therapist, Methodist Sports Medicine Center/The Orthopaedic Specialists, Indianapolis, Indiana

LISA CHINN, MS, ATC
PhD Candidate, University of Virginia, Exercise & Sport Injury Laboratory, Charlottesville, Virginia

JIM CLOVER, MED, ATC, PTA
Professor, Cal State San Bernardino; Instructor, Riverside Country Schools, The SPORT Clinic, Riverside, California

GEORGE J. DAVIES, DPT, MEd, SCS, ATC, CSCS
Professor of Physical Therapy, Armstrong Atlantic State University, Savannah, Georgia

TODD S. ELLENBECKER, DPT, MS, SCS, OCS, CSCS
Clinic Director, Physiotherapy Associates Scottsdale Sports Clinic; National Director of Clinical Research - Physiotherapy Associates, Director of Sports Medicine - ATP Tour, Scottsdale, Arizona

JAY HERTEL, PhD, ATC
Associate Professor of Kinesiology, University of Virginia, Exercise & Sport Injury Laboratory, Charlottesville, Virginia

VINCENT J. HUDSON, PhD, DPT, MBA, ATC
Chief Operating Officer, OAA Orthopaedic Specialists, Allentown, Pennsylvania

TAMERAH HUNT, PhD
Clinical Research Specialist, Assistant Professor of Clinical Allied Medical Professions, School of Allied Medical Professions, The Ohio State University, Columbus, Ohio

CARRIE A. JAWORSKI, MD
Director of Intercollegiate Sports Medicine & Head Team Physician, Northwestern University Department of Intercollegiate Sports Medicine, Evanston, Illinois; Assistant Professor of Family and Community Medicine, Northwestern University Feinberg School of Medicine, Chicago, Illinois

JEFF G. KONIN, PhD, ATC, PT
Associate Professor and Vice Chair, Department of Orthopaedics and Sports Medicine; Executive Director, Sports Medicine and Athletic Related Trauma (SMART) Institute, University of South Florida, Tampa, Florida

MICHELLE KRAUSE, PT, ATC
Director of Rehabilitation Services, Northwestern University Department of Intercollegiate Sports Medicine, Evanston, Illinois

TAD E. PIECZYNSKI, MS, PT, OCS, CSCS
Assistant Director, Physiotherapy Associates Scottsdale Sports Clinic, Scottsdale, Arizona

ERIC SAMPSELL, PT, ATC
Out-Patient Rehabilitation Coordinator, SMART Clinic Director, WVUH-East City Hospital, Foundation Way, Martinsburg, West Virginia

AIMEE A. SLATTERY, MS, PT, CSCS
PRO Sports PT, Scarsdale, New York

TIMOTHY F. TYLER, MS, PT, ATC
NISMAT at Lenox Hill Hospital, New York, New York

JEROME WALL, MD, FACS
The SPORT Clinic, Riverside, California

GREG WERNER, MS, MSCC, CSCS, SCCC, ACSM-HFI
Director of Strength and Conditioning Kinesiology; Faculty, James Madison University, Harrisonburg, Virginia

Contents

Rehabilitation plays an integral role when it comes to managing sports injuries in a safe and timely manner. Doing so competently allows for a greater chance of quick recovery and ultimate success on and off the field. Understanding the goals of rehabilitation and how to enhance communication between all providers who are involved with athlete care is critical to the process. The purpose of this article is to thoroughly explain the steps and critical components of a rehabilitation process designed specifically for each athlete's needs.

Sport-related concussions are becoming common place in athletics and daily activity. Proper assessment and management of concussions are crucial, as repeat concussion can result in prolonged symptoms and catastrophic outcomes. New research is changing the way concussions are managed. The previously used systems have been abandoned in favor of individualized assessment and management using a multidisciplinary approach to include clinical signs, neuropsychological assessment, and postural stability. Transitioning the new evidence to clinical practice is the future of diagnosis, management, and safe return to play following sport-related concussions. This article aims to bridge this gap and provide a systematic, easy-to-use methodology in the management of sport-related concussions.

The shoulder remains one of the more challenging joints for clinicians to clearly identify, diagnose, and treat within the athletic population. Its complexities involving the glenohumeral, acromioclavicular, sternoclavicular, and scapulothoracic joints moving in tandem require the physician and rehabilitation specialist to have a comprehensive understanding of the biomechanics and arthrokinematics associated with athletic activity. This chapter focuses on the evaluation, classification, mechanism of injury, and initial treatment of widespread shoulder injuries involved in sports.

Evaluation of the athlete with an elbow injury involves a complete upper extremity approach and a corresponding treatment approach that addresses the identified deficiencies to restore normal function. A significant focus should be placed on the proximal aspect of the upper extremity in addition to the obvious distal injury. A detailed review of the available treatment modalities fails to identify any clear definitive choice to address pain levels; however, a combination of modalities and appropriate exercise can be used in the early rehabilitation phases. The use of a total arm strengthening program along with evaluation of the athlete's sport mechanics is required to successfully return the patient back to their preinjury level of function. A supervised interval sport return program is also a necessary component of the complete rehabilitation program for the athlete with an elbow injury.

In sports, wrist and hand injuries are commonplace. Too often, injuries to these areas can be under-treated and left for further complications to arise. While some injuries to the wrist and hand can be treated conservatively with immediate return to play, others require a more in-depth assessment prior to return to play. This article describes the most common wrist and hand injuries in sport, and provides information related to current treatment approaches.

Rehabilitation of a knee injury is done in a criterion-based progression that is based on individual progress from one phase to another and not on a prespecified period of time. If the rehabilitation deviates from this approach, the body will react with adverse affects such as inflammation, pain, and further injury. Delay in the entire rehabilitation program will delay the athlete in meeting goals and returning to play. Phase I focuses on restoration of range of motion, pain modulation, inflammatory control, modification of activities, and gait training. Phase II is characterized by gaining full range of motion, demonstration of normal gait pattern, basic to advanced strengthening and flexibility, appropriate cardiovascular conditioning, and proprioception retraining. Phase III allows functional return to prior activity level. This phase includes a sport/occupational-specific functional progression. Utilizing a trained rehabilitation specialist will allow the athlete/individual an effective and efficient return to prior level of function.

An athlete often presents to the rehabilitation specialist with either a non-specific referral, such as "hip pain," or with a diagnosis of a more specific hip pathology. The highly skilled clinician is trained to look at the "linkage" between the trunk and all parts of the lower extremity. Why is the hip not transferring the load well? Where is the breakdown? The gluteus medius, pelvic stability, and supportive muscular slings are of great importance when optimizing the function of the hip. The hip is subjected to forces equal to multiples of the body weight and requires osseous, articular and myofascial integrity for stability. This is the mind set when devising an athlete's rehabilitative program, looking at all influential factors that affect joint movement and integrity.

The spine plays an essential role in the contribution toward athletic performance. As the central pillar of the body, the structures of the spine are susceptible to injury related with sports participation. This article identifies many of the most commonly seen sports-related injuries to the spine, and discusses practical rehabilitative interventions to manage such injuries. Anatomic considerations, biomechanical movements, and tissue properties are explained to better understand the clinical expectations associated with each of the injuries described.

Foot and ankle injuries are extremely common among athletes and other physically active individuals. Rehabilitation programs that emphasize the use of therapeutic exercise to restore joint range of motion, muscle strength, neuromuscular coordination, and gait mechanics have been shown to have clinical success for patients suffering various foot and ankle pathologies. Rehabilitation programs are discussed for ankle sprains, plantar fasciitis, Achilles tendonitis, and turf toe.

Determining the criteria for an injured athlete's return to competition can be a confusing scenario when all the individuals involved are brought in. These may include the athlete, parents, guardians, coaches, family physician, the athletic trainer, and others. Providing a foundation from which all can understand the reasoning is key. It must be understood that the primary responsibility is to cause no harm to the athlete, while enabling him or her to participate at the highest level possible. This article discusses the importance of establishing guidelines, athletes' behavioral responses

THE CLINICS ARE NOW AVAILABLE ONLINE!

Access your subscription at:
www.theclinics.com

Foreword

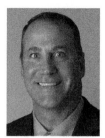

Mark D. Miller, MD
Consulting Editor

Well, Dr Konin has done it again! He has put together another stellar issue for the *Clinics in Sports Medicine* series. The concept here is for team physicians to appreciate what a certified athletic trainer expects and understands in order to work together as a team to optimize the care of athletes.

This issue does a nice job of including a variety of topics, from concussion management to detailed treatises on specific anatomic areas. Rehabilitation is heavily emphasized because it is an important part of successful athletic care. As we all know, a certified athletic trainer can often be the best "therapist" for this challenging population. Do not miss the article on return to play. This has been a popular subject for instructional course lectures in a variety of venues and is an important area that does not have a lot of published guidelines to help health care teams.

Jeff Konin is an outstanding trainer, administrator, editor, and author. My career has been richly rewarded through his teaching…now yours can be as well!

Mark D. Miller, MD
University of Virginia
400 Ray C. Hunt Drive
Suite 330, Charlottesville
VA 22908-0159, USA

E-mail address:
mdm3p@virginia.edu (M.D. Miller)

Clin Sports Med 29 (2010) xi
doi:10.1016/j.csm.2009.09.010
0278-5919/09/$ – see front matter © 2010 Elsevier Inc. All rights reserved.

Preface

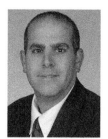

Jeff G. Konin, PhD, ATC, PT
Guest Editor

This issue of *Clinics in Sports Medicine* has been put together to provide practicing clinicians with current information regarding treatment interventions for today's athletes. Some of the leaders in the profession of sports medicine have gathered to contribute to this compilation of timely and relevant information. The management of athletes at all levels is constantly changing as effective outcomes are identified that lead to quicker and safer return to participation. In the space allotted, we chose what we thought are some of the common concerns affecting physicians, athletic trainers, physical therapists, and others who work closely with the athletic population.

The brainchild of this project is Mark Miller, MD, touted orthopedic surgeon at the University of Virginia, prolific writer in the area of sports medicine, and the series editor for *Clinics in Sports Medicine*. As the orthopedic team physician for James Madison University, Mark is an avid supporter of the role rehabilitation plays in the successful performance of athletes. He empowers those who design, implement, and supervise athletic rehabilitation programs and he truly believes in a collaborative teamwork approach to managing athletic injuries.

In this issue, evidence-based contemporary methods are conveyed to readers for common sports injuries of the shoulder, elbow, wrist and hand, spine, hip, knee, and ankle. In addition, an excellent summary of concussion assessment and management is provided that provides clarity for return-to-play guidelines based on the most recent findings related to head injuries. An article on strength and conditioning is included to demonstrate the importance of an interdisciplinary approach for athletes' care. Finally, to enhance effective communication between physicians and other health care providers, an article outlining the most effective ways to exchange referral-based information is included. This type of information oftentimes is left out of discussion in most publications yet it serves as one of the most important components for achieving beneficial results for athletic rehabilitation.

I hope that the readers enjoy what they read and appreciate the scientific content provided by the contributors. The practical delivery of the information has been

Clin Sports Med 29 (2010) xiii–xiv
doi:10.1016/j.csm.2009.09.009

intentionally written in a way to provide useful information that can be incorporated into clinical practice Monday morning!

Jeff G. Konin, PhD, ATC, PT
Department of Orthopaedics and Sports Medicine
University of South Florida
13220 USF Laureal Drive
MDF 5th Floor
Mail Code MDC 106
Tampa, FL 33612, USA

E-mail address:
jkonin@health.usf.edu (J.G. Konin)

Introduction to Rehabilitation

Jeff G. Konin, PhD, ATC, PT

KEYWORDS

• Rehabilitation • Referral • Sports medicine
• Treatment • Utilization

GOALS OF REHABILITATION

Rehabilitation from a sports-related injury can range from a one-time patient education encounter to a year of intense supervised exercises and healing. Regardless of the time and effort required, one of the main purposes of rehabilitation is to provide individuals with a best-effort approach to a quick and safe return to participation. In sports, such an outcome seems imperative and demanded by most athletes, coaches, parents, and stakeholders associated with the game.

Generally speaking, the restoration of preinjury function serves as a primary goal of any rehabilitation program. Realistically, however, many individuals will never return to a level equal to that of the preinjury state whereas others may actually establish improved strength, proprioception, and flexibility as the result of a rehabilitation program. Thus, all programs are person-specific and should be designed and monitored as such, keeping in mind the individual needs of each athlete.

Benefits of rehabilitation after an injury may include but are not limited to the following:

- Restoration of unrestricted and pain-free joint range of motion
- Restoration of functional strength
- Decrease or complete removal of abnormal sensation (pain or absence of sensation)
- Reduction or elimination of inflammation
- Improved proprioception
- Improved awareness of posture and core stability
- Improved gait pattern
- Enhanced awareness and education regarding current injury and prevention of future injuries
- Improved cardiovascular functioning

Department of Orthopaedics and Sports Medicine, Sports Medicine and Athletic Related Trauma (SMART) Institute, College of Medicine, University of South Florida, 13220 USF Laurel Drive, MDF 5th Floor, Mail Code MDC106, Tampa, FL 33612, USA
E-mail address: jkonin@health.usf.edu

Clin Sports Med 29 (2010) 1–4
doi:10.1016/j.csm.2009.09.001
0278-5919/09/$ – see front matter

To many, rehabilitation is perceived as a process that takes place only after sustaining an injury. In the eyes of rehabilitations specialists, injury prevention is also considered a part of rehabilitation, viewed as a proactive intervention that can minimize or reduce the number and severity of injuries. Unfortunately, to some, rehabilitation is often bypassed or not considered necessary. In such cases, even absent a single-patient educational interaction, athletes' return to participation may be delayed. Furthermore, the time when they do return to participation may not be optimal regarding being the most prepared for avoiding reinjury. Although perhaps biased, rehabilitation professionals support the notion of early intervention in all cases in an effort to reduce unnecessary side effects, complications, and patient unawareness of contraindications and precautions.

As an example, ample literature supports the notion that a minimal amount of joint swelling, although perhaps commonplace in many so called minor sports injuries, can have significant effects on functional abilities. Studies have shown that function may be hindered by joint inflammation as a result of limited range of motion, decrease in neuromuscular facilitation, and decreased muscular strength.[1-3]

REHABILITATION SPECIALIST

In the sports medicine setting, a cadre of individuals collaborates to form sports medicine teams. Arguably, educational training and advanced skill sets can be individualized to a single credential or profession. Additionally, some components of rehabilitation intervention overlap from one professional to another. This is seen regardless of the provider: physician, chiropractor, athletic trainer, physical therapist, and so forth. Ultimately, the provider of choice should be competent and current in a skill set, be appropriately licensed, and have a good understanding of working with the athletic population.

Rehabilitation specialists working with athletes must understand the physical and psychologic demands of sport. Despite what many say, an ankle sprain is not an ankle sprain. There is more than simply understanding the anatomy of the ligament torn and a few simple exercises that can be safely performed to restore function. Rehabilitation specialists working with athletes should be prepared in the following ways:

- Possess a clear understanding of a given sport that an athlete participates in
- Understand the biomechanics and pathomechanics of various sports
- Be familiar with protective equipment for various sports
- Understand the physiologic expectations of the sports
- Understand differences in youth versus adult sports-related injuries
- Keep abreast with injury prevention programs and return to play criteria (ie, anterior cruciate ligament injury prevention or return to play from a concussion)
- Know elements of preparticipation physical examinations
- Recognize disqualifications from sport criteria as they relate to organizations (National Collegiate Athletic Association and high school federations)
- Possess current emergency care qualifications and training

This list could continue for pages. Some rehabilitation specialists establish a focus and primary area of care. This might include postoperative rehabilitation, injury prevention, or emergency care. Regardless, they should possess competence and be prepared to work with a team approach for the most successful outcome afforded to any athlete.

THE REHABILITATION REFERRAL

Physicians have different philosophies and working relationships with rehabilitation specialists. These patterns are based on training experiences and perhaps even personal experiences with rehabilitation after their own orthopedic injury.

It is imperative for rehabilitation specialists and physicians to have a good working relationship, one that includes accessible communication and trust between each other. If physicians are ever in doubt as to whether or not an athlete should be referred for rehabilitation, a referral should always occur and allow for a rehabilitation specialist to determine the need for any intervention that could assist with a safe recovery. The same holds true for rehabilitation specialists who are uncertain if an athlete needs to be assessed by a physician—such a decision should always favor the athlete with an additional consultation that may prove valuable.

The communication between the two professionals should occur in a timely manner but more importantly should convey the necessary information to proceed with a plan to manage an athlete's injury. Despite the fact that inappropriate referrals may occur, a single consultation can do no harm if further intervention is not warranted. The examples discussed here focus on the referral information that should be provided by a physician to a rehabilitation specialist.

The mode of communication is secondary to the actual occurrence of the communication itself. The more that is placed in writing, however, the more information tends to be conveyed clearly from one party to another. Any standard protocols followed by either party should be communicated ahead of time in an effort to reduce the time to treatment intervention for an athlete and to implement agreed-on approaches in advance. Athletes, coaches, and parents tend to find a sense of comfort knowing that physicians and rehabilitation specialists have an existing relationship and understand each other's expectations.

The actual referral in written form typically occurs in the form of a script written by a physician. Such scripts may have little information conveyed, such as stating, "evaluate and treat," or they may be overly inclusive and state parameters that include, for instance, ultrasound delivery modes. Although there is no perfect referral, there are some guidelines that assist rehabilitation specialists with treatment interventions.[4] The following is a list of suggestions for physicians when communicating requests for rehabilitation of an athlete:

- Scripts with vague information will likely prompt a phone call—be thorough but not overly detailed.
- Scripts with excessive detail may not be appropriate. For example, stating specific parameters for ultrasound may be unwarranted, as these need to be modified at the time of treatment.
- Scripts should always contain essential information required for reimbursement purposes, to include but not limited to date, signature, diagnosis, and number and frequency of treatments. These may vary from state to state based on insurance carrier guidelines.
- Clearly communicate any critical contraindications, precautions, and timelines on the referral script.
- A correspondence from a rehabilitation specialist is usually an indication that an important piece of information needs to be conveyed. This may be something a physician needs to provide the therapist in order to proceed, or it may be an update by a therapist to receive assurance from the physician of the next phases. Return the call!

- Appoint a person in the office to serve as a liaison when you are seeing patients so that inquiries can be responded to in a timely manner.
- Keep in mind therapeutic modalities are an adjunct to manual intervention, exercise, and patient education. If you think a modality is warranted, it may be better to suggest this to the rehabilitation therapist as a possibility as opposed to a mandate stated on a referral. A statement, such as "modalities as needed," allows for flexibility in treatment intervention as symptoms change.

The bottom line is that the clearer the communication between a referring physician and a rehabilitation specialist, the more likely athletes will experience a positive outcome and a safe return to participation. A stronger relationship between providers often translates into improved communications.

The articles in this issue have been written by rehabilitation specialists and physicians in a collaborative effort to offer protocol-based approaches and critical thinking interventions using the most currently available evidence. The information has been condensed to provide readers with straightforward information as it pertains to the rehabilitation of various sports-related injuries.

REFERENCES

1. Palmieri RM, Ingersoll CD, Edwards JE, et al. Arthrogenic muscle inhibition is not present in the limb contralateral to a simulated knee joint effusion. Am J Phys Med Rehabil 2003;82(12):910–6.
2. Palmieri RM, Tom JA, Edwards JE, et al. Arthrogenic muscle response induced by an experimental knee joint effusion is mediated by pre- and post-synaptic spinal mechanisms. J Electromyogr Kinesiol 2004;14(6):631–40.
3. Palmieri RM, Weltman A, Edwards JE, et al. Pre-synaptic modulation of quadriceps arthrogenic muscle inhibition. Knee Surg Sports Traumatol Arthrosc 2005;13(5): 370–6.
4. Rand SE, Goerlich C, Marchand K, et al. The physical therapy prescription [review]. Am Fam Physician 2007;76(11):1661–6.

Concussion Assessment and Management

Tamerah Hunt, PhD[a],*, Chad Asplund, MD[b]

KEYWORDS

- Concussion • Head injury • Athletic training
- Assessment • Management

Sport-related concussion is a common injury in athletes. However, it is frequently underreported, which makes the diagnosis a challenge. The management of sport-related concussions has changed significantly over the last several years. The previously used grading systems and return-to-play guidelines have been abandoned in favor of more individualized assessment and management. A multidisciplinary approach, including neuropsychological testing, is being used more frequently to assist in management. After recovery, it is recommended that athletes' return-to-play progress is in a gradual, stepwise fashion while being monitored by a health care provider.

Concussions have reached near-epidemic proportions in contact sports at professional and amateur levels; there are an estimated 1.6 to 3.8 million sport-related concussions occurring in the United States annually.[1] The effects of a concussion can have severe negative effects on athletes' scholastic abilities and can sometimes end a career.

Proper assessment and management of a sport-related concussion is crucial, as repeat concussions can result in decreased neurocognitive functioning, increased symptomatology, and at times, catastrophic outcomes. Recently, there has been an abundance of research in an effort to better define, diagnose, manage, and treat concussion. Bridging the gap between research and clinical practice is the key to reducing the incidence and severity of sport-related concussion and improving return-to-play decisions. The purpose of this article is to discuss the current evidence available to assist practitioners in the diagnosis and management of concussion to ensure safe participation for all athletes.

DEFINITION

Sports-related concussion appears to result in transient symptoms with short duration. There are no universal agreements on the definition of concussion. The most

[a] School of Allied Medical Professions, The Ohio State University, 2050 Kenny Road Suite 3100, Columbus, OH 43221, USA
[b] Department of Family Medicine, Division of Sports Medicine, The Ohio State University, 2050 Kenny Road, Suite 3100, Columbus, OH 43221, USA
* Corresponding author.
E-mail address: tamerah.hunt@osumc.edu (T. Hunt).

Clin Sports Med 29 (2010) 5–17
doi:10.1016/j.csm.2009.09.002

commonly accepted and cited definition is based on functional status and the nature of medical signs and symptoms present at the time of injury.

Concussion has been defined as "a complex pathophysiological process affecting the brain, induced by traumatic biomechanical forces."[2,3] This consensus from the First and Third International Conference for Concussion suggested five conditions for concussion:

1. Concussion may be caused either by a direct blow to the head, face, neck, or elsewhere on the body with an impulsive or rotational force transmitted to the head.
2. Concussion typically results in the rapid onset of short-lived impairment of neurologic function that resolves spontaneously.
3. Concussion may result in neuropathologic changes, but the acute clinical symptoms rarely reflect a functional disturbance rather than structural injury.
4. Concussion results in a graded set of clinical syndromes that may or may not involve loss of consciousness; resolution of the clinical and cognitive symptoms typically follows a sequential course.
5. Concussion is typically associated with grossly normal structural neuroimaging studies.

This accepted definition has changed the evaluation techniques and management of sports-related concussion for many medical professionals.

COMMONLY USED EVALUATION TOOLS

Recently, several agencies have produced position and consensus statements suggesting a multifaceted approach to assessment and management of concussion.[4–6] The multifaceted approach captures the variability of deficits following injury. The recent addition of neuropsychological and balance assessment to the concussion assessment battery provides the clinician with additional information specific to areas commonly associated with concussion. The concussion assessment battery begins with physical evaluation and may contain imaging, self-reported symptoms, and sideline assessments; neuropsychological and postural testing provides the most comprehensive test battery for individualized concussion assessment.

Physical Evaluation

Physical evaluation typically occurs on the sideline or within the first few minutes of injury. When surveyed, more than 85% of physicians used the clinical examination as the primary assessment tool for concussion. Although physical examination is typically the first line of assessment, it is often combined with additional concussion assessment tools.[7] The physical evaluation typically includes a complete history and an evaluation of nervous, motor, and sensory systems following injury.

A complete history provides information regarding the likelihood of previous concussion, symptoms occurring not related to current concussive injury, or post-concussive symptoms. Nervous evaluation typically consists of cranial nerve assessment with special emphasis on pupillary reflex. Motor system evaluation includes myotome strength testing for tone and ability with special emphasis on the cervical region and areas distal to the injury. Sensory assessment involves evaluation of dull and sharp sensation, bilateral sensation, and dermatome testing.

Imaging

The hallmark of sports-related concussion presents with functional deficits rather than structural deficits. There is good evidence that imaging techniques such as X ray, MRI, and CT would be unable to detect concussion unless there were gross structural changes in the brain.[2] CT and traditional MRI, therefore, may not be as useful as initially thought. Newer technologies may offer different techniques to evaluate brain function using imaging.

Functional MRI (fMRI) provides information regarding neural function during task performance using a noninvasive technique.[8,9] fMRI has been used with dual task paradigms in concussion assessment.[10] Other techniques include magnetic source imaging (MSI), which uses MRI to obtain anatomic information while investigating the electrophysiology data from magnetoencephalography.[9,11] MSI offers tracking of real-time brain activity, without distorting, by conduction through the brain, skull, and scalp.

The metabolic changes post concussion suggests the use of positron emission tomography (PET) and single-photon emission CT (SPECT), which evaluates metabolism of the specified region and blood flow (respectively) associated with activation of that region.[8,9,11] These measures attempt to quantify correlations between metabolic flow and injury severity, post-concussion symptoms, and recovery.[11]

As technology continues to improve, understanding the effects and consequences of concussion should also improve. Newer techniques are currently only available to researchers because of cost, availability, and accessibility. Use of X ray, MRI, and CT scan may be helpful in identifying life-threatening injuries and should be used as a precaution when fMRI, MSI, PET, and SPECT scans are not available. If imaging is not possible, continual monitoring of symptoms and patients' condition can provide useful information post concussion.

Self-Report Symptoms

Interactions between medical professionals and athletes are commonly completed by athlete self-report of symptoms. Several self-report symptom scales and checklists exist to quantify symptom severity and duration. Common scales are the Post Concussion Symptom Scale, the Graded Symptom Checklist, and the Head Injury Scale. When surveyed, 85% of certified athletic trainers used symptom checklists as part of concussion assessment battery.[7]

Several symptoms have been linked to the occurrence of concussion. These symptoms can be divided into somatic, cognitive, and sensory domains.[12] These include somatic symptoms such as headache, nausea, and vomiting; cognitive symptoms to include memory loss and slowed thinking; and sensory symptoms such as fatigue, drowsiness, and difficulty sleeping. Concussed athletes exhibit an increase in symptoms reported acutely, but follow a nonlinear recovery.[13–15] Baseline assessment is valuable in symptom assessment as several investigators found that athletes self-report the presence of symptoms during baseline testing.[12,16] Although attention must be paid to concussion-related symptoms that naturally occur, such as headache, the intensity and frequency of these symptoms will increase following concussion. Reliable self-reports are dependent upon the interaction between athlete and medical professional and the desire for the athlete to return to participation. Clinicians should take caution when relying solely on athletes' self report alone, the use of a multifaceted approach is still highly recommended.

Sideline Assessments

Acutely, a concussed individual may display transient changes in cognition, postural ability, and symptom reports. The ability to obtain a measure of these deficits immediately following injury provides invaluable information for the occurrence and management of concussion. The most commonly used sideline assessment is the Standardized Assessment of Concussion (SAC), and more recently, the Sport Concussion Assessment Tool (SCAT).

The SAC is a neurocognitive examination that was specifically intended for the assessment of athletes who have concussions on the sideline of play. The test components include orientation, memory, concentration, and delayed recall. Athletes who had concussion scored significantly different than athletes who did not, with scores 48 hours post-injury returning to baseline values for the injured group.[17] A decline in SAC score at the time of injury is 95% sensitive and 76% specific in accurately classifying injured and uninjured subjects. Reliability analysis demonstrated that test-retest reliability of 0.53.[17]

The SCAT was developed as a part of the Summary and Agreement Statement of the Second International Symposium on Concussion. The SCAT is a compilation of tools commonly used by sports medicine professionals. It includes a concussion symptom checklist, concentration and memory tasks, and neurologic screening; however, reliability and validity evidence is unavailable at this time.

Neuropsychological Tests

Recently, neuropsychological tests have gained favor in the profession of athletic training as tools for assessing cognitive function before and following concussion. Neuropsychological testing is used to provide a sensitive index of higher brain functioning by measuring functions such as memory, attention, executive function, and speed and flexibility of cognitive processing. These functions have been determined to become sensitive during impairments associated with concussion.

Commonly used pencil and paper tests include Trail Making Test,[13,18,19] Digit Symbol Substitution Test,[13,20] Controlled Oral Word Association Test, Hopkins Verbal Learning Test, and the Stroop Word Color Test.[19] Several computerized neuropsychological platforms have recently been developed and include the Automated Neuropsychological Assessment Metrics, Cogsport, Headminder, and Immediate Post-Assessment of Concussion Test.[21–24] These platforms boost higher sensitivity and more accurate measures of reaction time. Further, the computerized battery can be administered in small groups with no loss of reliability.

A significant amount of evidence supports the use of neuropsychological testing following concussion. The evidence suggests that recovery patterns for collegiate and professional athletes following concussion lasts from hours[13,25] up to 7 days.[14,19] Following a concussive injury, individuals typically display transient deficits in cognitive functioning that can often be detected through neuropsychological assessment.

Although these tests are considered to be the gold standard in concussion assessment, they have never been validated for use with concussed athletes.[26] Further, there has been no consensus among researchers as to which neuropsychological tests within the battery are the most sensitive in detecting change following concussion.[27]

Posturography

Following concussive injuries, athletes may have difficultly integrating information from the three components of the balance mechanism. Although the somatosensory aspect appears to remain normal, integration between the visual and vestibular components does not function properly.[19]

The two most commonly used postural assessments are the Neurocom Sensory Organization Test and the Balance Error Scoring System (BESS). The Sensory Organization Test (SOT) within the Neurocom Smart Balance Master uses a force plate that has the ability to measure angles and forces being generated at the ankle, knee, and hip. The test systematically alters visual and somatosensory referencing in an attempt to individually evaluate the three components of the balance mechanism (visual, vestibular, and somatosensory). The SOT is the gold standard for postural stability in concussion; however, the SOT is not portable and is very expensive.

The BESS was developed as an objective assessment tool to be used by clinicians with minimal cost and training for the evaluation of postural stability following concussion. Athletes who have a concussion have shown deficits in postural stability using the SOT and BESS for up to 5 days postinjury in a collegiate population with recovery to pre-injury values usually occurring within 4 to 7 days. Postural assessment within a concussion battery has been evidenced as postural deficits following injury were present after symptoms resolution and cognitive deficits dissipated.[19,28]

Concussion assessment tools are recommended in combination to obtain the most complete information regarding deficits post-concussion. Broglio and colleagues[29] found that neuropsychological testing in combination with self-reported symptoms produces a sensitivity of 89% to 96% following concussion. As the deficits following concussion carry the same variability as the individuals who have concussions, a multifaceted approach provides information regarding as many deficit areas as possible. Obtaining the most information possible will enable clinicians to offer quality care and management while providing good, reliable, and safe return-to-participation decisions.

TREATMENT OPTIONS

When faced with a sports-related concussion, the provider may ask, "What treatments are available?" There are no specific medical therapies for concussion. Most patients improve with education, cognitive rest, and time for the brain to recover.

Pharmacologic treatment in sports concussion may be applied in two distinct situations: (1) management of specific symptoms (ie, sleep disturbance, anxiety) and (2) to modify the underlying pathophysiology of the condition with the aim of shortening the duration of the concussion symptomatology. Pharmacologic therapies should only be used by those providers with training and experience in managing concussion.[3] Although there are no specific treatments, the following therapies have been studied and the evidence is presented.

Educational Interventions

To date, the strongest evidence is in support of the effectiveness of early patient-education initiatives.[30] There is good evidence to endorse the notion that supportive patient-centered interaction and the provision of symptom-related education by practitioners is effective in assisting individuals to recover from concussion symptoms. Studies show that most patients respond best to appropriate information and reassurance.[31,32]

Neurocognitive Rehabilitation

Neurocognitive rehabilitation, which mainly focuses on treating specific individualized cognitive deficits, is one of the most widely used treatments for severe brain injury,[33] but there is no conclusive evidence supporting improved outcome in mild traumatic brain injury or concussion. Studies, however, have demonstrated improvement in neuropsychological testing following neurocognitive rehabilitation, but there is some debate over whether this was because of a practice effect, which may have artificially raised scores.[34]

Pharmacologic Interventions

Pharmacologic treatment in sports concussion may be considered in the management of specific symptoms or in an attempt to modify the underlying pathophysiology of the condition with the aim of shortening the duration of the concussion symptomatology.[35] The most common symptom for which treatment is indicated is the post-concussion headache.[36] However, the results of studies of the efficacy of pharmacologic therapy have not been promising.

There are many pharmacologic management options that have been proposed for all grades of brain injury, but in many cases, the evidence is based upon studies of severe brain injury and the results may not be directly applicable to concussion. Also, a recent systematic review of pharmacologic interventions after minor traumatic brain injury failed to produce solid evidence that any specific drug treatment is effective for one or more symptoms of mild traumatic brain injury.[34]

Amitriptyline

The evidence is conflicting regarding the effectiveness of amitriptyline as a treatment for persistent post concussion headache. A case series found that amitriptyline may be effective in doses from 75 to 225 mg/d,[37] whereas a more rigorous clinical trial found no benefit for amitriptyline.[38]

Corticosteroids

Corticosteroids have been used in the past, presumably based on their ability to stabilize membranes and reduce inflammation. However, a systematic review of randomized controlled trials of corticosteroids in acute traumatic brain injury shows that there remains considerable uncertainty over their effects. Neither moderate benefits nor moderate harmful effects can be excluded.[39]

Free Radical Scavengers and Antioxidants

Antioxidant therapies provide numerous beneficial and protective effects following injury in animal models involving physical, cognitive, and affective issues. To date, no human trial performed so far has successfully demonstrated efficacy.[40] Also, there is some concern raised by the large epidemiologic studies of antioxidant use for cardiovascular disease where antioxidant therapy was associated with an increase in cancer incidence.

Non-steroidal Antiinflammatory Drugs

Toxic breakdown products of arachidonic acid metabolism have been hypothesized to exacerbate central nervous system injury. Studies of cyclooxygenase inhibitors (eg, ibuprofen) and mixed cyclooxygenase-lipoxygenase inhibitors have shown some therapeutic benefit in animal models of spinal cord injury, but no specific trials of this therapy have been performed with mild traumatic brain injury.[41]

Calcium Channel Antagonists

The entry of calcium through voltage-dependent channels may contribute to secondary brain injury. Despite the intuitive logic of treatment with calcium channel antagonists, several randomized trials of various agents have failed to demonstrate protective benefits.[42,43]

Nicotinamide

Nicotinamide (Vitamin B3) is a potent neuroprotectant following brain injury in animals.[44] Administration of Vitamin B3 following head injury has also been shown to improve functional recovery in injured rats.[45] Although early administration of Vitamin B3 is promising, it is unclear if this will translate to humans following concussion.

Hyperbaric Oxygen Therapy

The delivery of high concentrations of oxygen under pressure has been proposed as a means of enhancing cerebral oxygenation, and hence, injury recovery post-concussion. Possible mechanisms of action include cerebral vasoconstriction, improvement in glucose metabolism, and reduction of cerebral edema. However, hyperbaric oxygen may also have a potentially harmful effect by increasing oxygen supply for free radical reactions. In severe brain injuries, randomized trials have demonstrated an improved mortality rate with hyperbaric therapy; however, there was no improvement in functional outcome at 12 months.[46]

RETURN-TO-PLAY CRITERIA FOLLOWING A CONCUSSION

Each concussion is as individual as the athletes that sustain them, and moreover, every return-to-play criteria varies from institution to institution. The variation typically depends on the training of the medical staff, the tools available to the medical staff, and the relationship that members of the medical staff have with their athletes, coaches, and administration.

A sound plan between all members of the medical team should be agreed upon before any competitive season. The team physician should drive the protocol through a collaborative decision-making process with everyone (athletic trainers, physical therapists, and other allied medical professionals) involved. The team physician should lead this team of professionals by providing information and concurring with the plan of action to ensure continuity of management following a concussive injury.

Recent guidelines suggest a multifaceted approach to concussion assessment to capture the variability of deficits following injury. These guidelines are accompanied by the suggestion of baseline testing all athletes before the competitive season to compare pre-morbid function with that of post-injury. Neuropsychological tests for sports-related concussions can be administered before injury. Pretesting provides a baseline to the medical staff who are evaluating athletes post injury so that subtle changes in cognitive and motor function can be detected. Pretesting would allow for a direct comparison of normal, should athletes become injured. In the event that baseline scores are not available, clinicians should use published norms accounting for any comorbidities that may affect testing, such as learning disabilities, previous history of concussion, medication usage, and mental conditions.

The clinical paradigm for your institution should include some type of cognitive assessment (preferably neuropsychological testing), balance testing, and a self-report symptom assessment (**Fig. 1**). All testing should be completed once the athlete is asymptomatic. Testing while the athlete is symptomatic does not provide additional information and typically encourages practice effects. Further, clinical utility of testing while symptomatic is nonsense as return to participation would not be a safe and practical option.

Several return-to-play criteria have been developed. Previously, return-to-play paradigms were based upon anecdotal evidence and symptom resolution. Today, research provides tools that should be used to evaluate athletes' readiness for return. These guidelines are still based upon symptom resolution; however, additional tools are included in evaluation and return to play to avoid premature return to play and potential secondary injury (**Box 1**).

Individuals who have a suspected concussion must not be permitted to resume contact or regular activity until they can move with usual dexterity and speed and are perfectly oriented as to the time, place, their own identity,[47] and are able to identify the activities in which they were engaged just before the injury.[48] Each institution can develop their own return-to-play protocols, however the protocol should be a graduated, step-wise protocol with a return to rest upon the presence of symptoms.[3] Further, return-to-play protocols can be extended to fit the severity and duration of initial cognitive symptoms (**Box 2**).

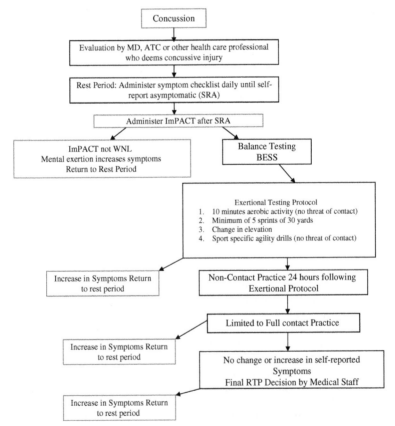

Fig. 1. The Ohio State University Sports Medical Center clinical paradigm.

Box 1
The Ohio State University Sports Medical Center's standard return-to-play exertional protocols

Standard Return to Play

Day 1

   30 to 40 minutes of nonimpact aerobic activity

      Exercise bike 15 minutes up to heart rate of 120 beats per minute (bpm)

      Cool down for 5 minutes

      Increase intensity, maximum heart rate of 145 to150 bpm, maintain for 15 minutes

      Cool down for 5 minutes

   No additional physical exertion

Immediately discontinue activity if there is any increase in athletes' symptoms and return to rest without physical activity until symptoms resolve.
Day 2

45 minutes of aerobic activity including jogging, running, sprints, or position-specific athletic drills; no contact

   Cool down for 5 minutes

   After at least 30 minutes rest, may lift weights for 30 minutes

Immediately discontinue activity if there is any increase in athletes' symptoms and return to rest without physical activity until symptoms resolve.

Day 3

   Full participation practice

Immediately discontinue activity if there is any increase in athletes' symptoms and return to rest without physical activity until symptoms resolve.

Day 4

   Full game participation

PRECAUTIONS AND RECOMMENDATIONS

During rehabilitation or follow-up, the referring physician should be aware of signs and symptoms of worsening conditions. Further, the physician should caution all of those involved with the rehabilitation process regarding stipulations following a concussive injury. This may include strength and conditioning coaches, academic advisors, and others that have interaction with athletes who have concussions. If athletes report an increase in symptoms, the medical professional should decrease cognitive and physical exertion. Further stipulations include

- symptoms increasing with mental and physical exertion
- mental status changes
- worsening strength deficits

FUTURE AREAS OF RESEARCH/INTEREST

We continually seek the one test that will determine the occurrence of a concussive injury, and how many concussive injuries are too many. These questions haunt the best

Box 2
The Ohio State University Sports Medical Center's extended return-to-play exertional protocols

Extended 5-Day Return to Play

Day 1

    30 to 40 minutes of nonimpact aerobic activity

    Exercise bike 15 minutes up to heart rate of 120 bpm

    Cool down for 5 minutes

    Increase intensity, maximum heart rate of 145 to150 bpm, maintain for 15 minutes

    Cool down for 5 minutes

    No additional physical exertion

Immediately discontinue activity if there is any increase in athletes' symptoms and return to rest without physical activity until symptoms resolve.

Day 2

    30 to 40 minutes of nonimpact aerobic activity

    Exercise bike 10 minutes up to heart rate of 120 bpm

    Cool down for 5 minutes

    Increase intensity, maximum heart rate of 145 to150 bpm, maintain for 25 minutes

    Cool down for 5 minutes

    No additional physical exertion

Immediately discontinue activity if there is any increase in athletes' symptoms and return to rest without physical activity until symptoms resolve.

Day 3

    45 minutes of aerobic activity including jogging, running, sprints, or position-specific athletic drills; no contact

    Cool down for 5 minutes

    After at least 30 minute rest may lift weights for 30 minutes

Immediately discontinue activity if there is any increase in athletes' symptoms and return to rest without physical activity until symptoms resolve.

Day 4

    Full participation practice

Immediately discontinue activity if there is any increase in athletes' symptoms and return to rest without physical activity until symptoms resolve.

Day 5

    Full game participation

researchers; however, other questions are revolving and evolving all aspects of concussion assessment and management. These questions resolve around the following

- The effects of comorbidities in concussion assessment and management
- Predisposing factors associated with incidence of concussion
- Educational interventions and the prevention of secondary injury

- Objective testing for the diagnosis of concussion featuring newer technologies
- Rehabilitative techniques and tools that may be used with concussion with the increase of technological improvement

REFERENCES

1. Langlois JA, Rutland-Brown W, Wald MM. The epidemiology and impact of traumatic brain injury: a brief overview. J Head Trauma Rehabil 2006;21:375–8.
2. Aubry M, Cantu R, Dvorak J, et al. Summary and agreement statement of the First International Conference on Concussion in Sport, Vienna 2001. Recommendations for the improvement of safety and health of athletes who may suffer concussive injuries. Br J Sports Med 2002;36(1):6–10.
3. McCrory P, Meeuwise W, Johnston K, et al. Consensus statement on concussion in sport- the 3rd International Conference on Concussion in Sport held in Zurich, November 2008. J Sci Med Sport 2009;12:340–51.
4. Guskiewicz KM, Bruce S, Cantu R, et al. National Athletic Trainers' Association position statement: management of sport-related concussion. J Athl Train 2004; 39(3):280–97.
5. McCrory P, Johnston K, Meeuwisse W, et al. Summary and agreement statement of the 2nd International Conference on Concussion in Sport, Prague 2004. Br J Sports Med 2005;39:196–204.
6. Herring S, Bergfield J, Boland A, et al. Concussion (mild traumatic brain injury) and the team physician: a consensus statement. Med Sci Sports Exerc 2006; 38(2):395–9.
7. Notebaert AJ, Guskiewicz KM. Current trends in athletic training practice for concussion assessment and management. J Athl Train 2005;40(4):320–35.
8. Bazarian JJ, Blyth B, Cimpello L. Bench to bedside: evidence for brain injury after concussion- looking beyond the computed tomography scan. Acad Emerg Med 2006;13:199–214.
9. Mendez CV, Hurley RA, Lassonde M, et al. Mild traumatic brain injury: neuroimaging of sports-related concussion. J Neuropsychiatry Clin Neurosci 2005;17(3):297–303.
10. Broglio SP, Tomporowski PD, Ferrara MS. Balance performance with a cognitive task: a dual task testing paradigm. Med Sci Sports Exerc 2005;37(4):689–95.
11. McAllister TW, Sparling MB, Flashman LA, et al. Neuroimaging findings in mild traumatic brain injury. J Clin Exp Neuropsychol 2001;23(6):775–91.
12. Piland SG, Motl RW, Ferrara MS, et al. Evidence for the factorial and construct validity of a self-report concussion symptom scale. J Athl Train 2003;38(2):104–12.
13. Macciocchi SN, Barth JT, Alves W, et al. Neuropsychological functioning and recovery after mild head injury in collegiate athletes. Neurosurgery 1996;39(3): 510–4.
14. McCrea M, Guskiewicz KM, Marshall SW, et al. Acute effects and recovery time following concussion in collegiate football players: the NCAA Concussion Study. JAMA 2003;290:2556–63.
15. Guskiewicz KM, McCrea M, Marshall SW, et al. Cumulative effects associated with recurrent concussion in collegiate football players. The NCAA Concussion Study. JAMA 2003;290(19):2549–56.
16. Field M, Collins MW, Lovell MR, et al. Does age play a role in recovery from sports-related concussion? A comparison of high school and collegiate athletes. J Pediatr 2003;142(5):546–53.
17. McCrea M. Standardized mental status assessment of sports concussion. Clin J Sport Med 2001;11(3):176–81.

18. Guskiewicz KM, Riemann BL, Perrin DH, et al. Alternative approaches to the assessment of mild head injury in athletes. Med Sci Sports Exerc 1997;29(Suppl 7):S213–21.
19. Guskiewicz KM, Ross SE, Marshall SW. Postural stability and neuropsychological deficits after concussion in collegiate athletes. J Athl Train 2001;36(3): 263–73.
20. Maddocks D, Saling M. Neuropsychological deficits following concussion. Brain Inj 1996;10(2):99–103.
21. Collins MW, Iverson GL, Lovell MR, et al. On-field predictors of neuropsychological and symptom deficit following sports-related concussion. Clin J Sport Med 2003;13(4):222–9.
22. Collie A, Makdissi M, Maruff P, et al. Cognition in the days following concussion: comparison of symptomatic versus asymptomatic athletes. J Neurol Neurosurg Psychiatr 2006;77:241–5.
23. Erlanger D, Feldman D, Kutner K, et al. Development and validation of a web-based neuropsychological test protocol for sports-related return-to-play decision making. Arch Clin Neuropsychol 2003;18:293–316.
24. Bleiberg J, Cernich AN, Cameron K, et al. Duration of cognitive impairment after sports concussion. Neurosurgery 2005;54:1073–8.
25. Echemendia RJ, Putukian M, Mackin RS, et al. Neuropsychological test performance prior to and following sports-related mild traumatic brain injury. Clin J Sport Med 2001;11(1):23–31.
26. Grindel SH, Lovell MR, Collins MW. The assessment of sport-related concussion: the evidence behind neuropsychological testing and management. Clin J Sport Med 2001;11:134–43.
27. Randolph C, McCrea M, Barr W. Is neuropsychological testing useful in the management of sport-related concussion? J Athl Train 2005;40(3):139–52.
28. Thompson J, Sebastianelli W, Slobounov S. EEG and postural correlates of mild traumatic brain injury in athletes. Neurosci Lett 2005;377:158–63.
29. Broglio SP, Macciocchi SN, Ferrara MS. Sensitivity of the concussion assessment battery. Neurosurgery 2007;60:1050–8.
30. Wade DI, King NS, Wenden FJ, et al. Routine follow up after head injury: a second randomised controlled trial. J Neurol Neurosurg Psychiatr 1998;65:177–83.
31. King NS, Crawford S, Wenden FJ, et al. Interventions and service need following mild and moderate head injury: the Oxford Head Injury Service. Clin Rehabil 1997;11:13–27.
32. Mittenberg W, Canyock EM, Condit D, et al. Treatment of post-concussion syndrome following mild head injury. J Clin Exp Neuropsychol 2001;23:829–36.
33. Ho MR, Bennett TL. Efficacy of neuropsychological rehabilitation for mild-moderate traumatic brain injury. Arch Clin Neuropsychol 1997;12:1–11.
34. Comper P, Bisschop SM, Carnide N, et al. A systematic review of treatments for mild traumatic brain injury. Brain Inj 2005;19(11):863–80.
35. McCrory P. Should we treat concussion pharmacologically? Br J Sports Med 2002;36:3–6.
36. Solomon S. Post-traumatic headache. Med Clin North Am 2001;85:987–96, vii–viii.
37. Saran A. Antidepressants not effective in headache associated with minor closed head injury. Int J Psychiatry Med 1088;18:75–83.
38. Tyler GS, McNeely HE, Dick ML. Treatment of post-traumatic headache with amitryptiline. Headache 1980;20:213–6.
39. Alberson P, Roberts I. Corticosteroids in acute traumatic brain injury: systematic review of randomised controlled trials. BMJ 1997:314:1855.

40. Rigg JL, Elovic EP, Greenwald BD. A review of the effectiveness of antioxidant therapy to reduce neuronal damage in acute traumatic brain injury. J Head Trauma Rehabil 2005;20(4):389–91.
41. Hallenbeck J, Jacobs T, Faden A. Combined PGI2, indomethacin and heparin improves neurological recovery after spinal trauma in cats. J Neurosurg 1983; 58:749–54.
42. Teasdale G. A randomised trial of nimodipine in severe head injury. J Neurotrauma 1991;9:S545–50.
43. Compton J, Lee T, Jones N. A double blind placebo controlled trial of the calcium entry blocking drug nicardipine in the treatment of vasospasm following severe head injury. Br J Neurosurg 1990;4:9–16.
44. Maiese K, Chong ZZ. Nicotinamide: necessary nutrient emerges as a novel cytoprotectant for the brain. Trends Pharmacol Sci 2003;24(5):228–32.
45. Hoane MR, Akstulewicz SL, Toppen J. Treatment with vitamin B_3 improves functional recovery and reduces GFAP expression following traumatic brain injury in the rat. J Neurotrauma 2003;20(11):1189–99.
46. Rockswold G, Ford S, Anderson D. Results of a prospective randomised trial for the treatment of severely brain injured patients with hyperbaric oxygen. Neurosurgery 1992;76:929–34.
47. Maroon JC, Steele PB, Berlin R. Football head and neck injuries: an update. Clin Neurosurg 1980;27:414–24.
48. Yarnell PR, Lynch S. The "ding" amnestic states in football trauma. Neurology 1973;23:196–7.

Evaluation, Diagnosis, and Treatment of Shoulder Injuries in Athletes

Vincent J. Hudson, PhD, DPT, MBA, ATC

KEYWORDS

• Glenoid • Labrum • Rotator culff • Dislocation • Impingement

The shoulder complex and the goal to maintain its normal kinematic function remain among the greater challenges in sports medicine today. Consisting of four joints and a plethora of ligaments and muscles, the complex must move with the synergy and coordination similar to that of mechanical robotics, performing movement with graceful fluidity. Any variation of force, mobility, strength, stability, and flexibility within the shoulder complex will alter the function, yielding potential microtraumatic episodes, leading to failure and breakdown.

The glenohumeral joint alone has the capacity to have the humerus placed in over 16,000 positions differentiated by a single degree.[1] This amount of mobility, working in conjunction with the scapulothoracic, acromioclavicular (AC), and sternoclavicular joints, creates a synergy of kinematics that is found nowhere else within the body. The freedom of movement requires a unique pattern of stabilization throughout the necessary arcs of motion. These relationships allow for extreme functional mobility, with dramatic activity of daily living capabilities and equal mechanical challenges for the physically active on the playing field.

The importance of understanding the biomechanical complexities involved in normal shoulder function allows the clinician to evaluate, diagnose, and properly address the alterations and self-imposed functional changes of the shoulder complex with regard to normal patterned movement. Many times, the clinician will be required to address a multitude of mechanical issues unscrupulously involving related joints both directly and indirectly.

The initial phase of any biomechanical assessment regarding potential injury includes the ability to prevent injury before it occurs or manifests into a functional disability. In doing so, skilled evaluation of mechanics regarding athletic function of the shoulder complex through screening, both static and dynamic, could be used as an initial

OAA Orthopaedic Specialists, 250 Cetronia Road, Allentown, PA 18104, USA
E-mail address: vhudson@oaainstitute.com

Clin Sports Med 29 (2010) 19–32
doi:10.1016/j.csm.2009.09.003
0278-5919/09/$ – see front matter © 2010 Elsevier Inc. All rights reserved.

pre-emptive injury prevention technique. Specifically, shoulder motion requires significant angular rotation at each of the four shoulder joints during shoulder elevation.[2]

Unfortunately, the athletic population often develops inequalities in strength, muscular development, and proper and efficient kinematics long before the medical profession has an opportunity to intervene. Success in the early stages of a career often leads to overutilization, creating biomechanical and kinematic inadequacies that lead to long-term microtrauma, which often is overlooked at the risk of missing an opportunity to play. The cycle develops where poor mechanics lead to compensatory changes, which eventually snowball the microtraumatic sequence, thereby leading to the necessity of medical intervention.

The compensatory changes from normal shoulder mechanics also give rise to muscle fatigue considerably earlier during activity than those observed in the mechanically sound shoulder. The mechanisms that cause fatigue are specific to the tasks being performed.[3] In effect, those tasks that require shoulder-stabilizing muscles to work inefficiently, or outside the realm of the muscles primary function, yield to mechanical defect over periods of overuse and inappropriate muscle-stabilizing expectation.

Additionally, the intervention of present-day sports performance coaches, various conditioning gurus, and personal fitness coaches may promote general imbalances in the normal mechanics relating to shoulder function and its relationship to the sport-specific requirements. The well-intentioned exercise protocol can become the root of early-phase biomechanical alterations yielding to microtraumatic episode in many cases of youth and teen injury. The bench press, military press, and other various weight training exercises could promote those diagnoses discussed within this article. The assumption that a younger shoulder has no defects falls short of reality in today's adolescent athletic population.[4] Clinicians evaluating more experienced overhead athletes need to recognize that scapular posture asymmetry in unilateral overhead athletes may be considered normal.[5]

By developing a philosophy of skillful and thorough evaluation technique and the ability to recognize the multitude of mechanic differences, alterations, and compensatory modifications in normal shoulder complex motion, one can become astute in preventing, diagnosing, and rehabilitating a whole host of injuries and mechanical defects to the shoulder complex.

EVALUATION

The evaluation processes associated with the shoulder vary from other joint evaluations primarily because of anatomic considerations that perpetuate relative stability from associated joints. A prime example would be an athlete's inability to actively elevate the shoulder, demonstrating decreased range of motion (ROM) at the glenohumeral joint, primarily because of the laxity at the AC joint following an AC separation.

The evaluative processes should include mechanism of injury, related past medical history, and notable deficits in ROM, strength and stability, anatomic sensitive structures upon palpation, neurologic involvement, and functional limitations. The development of a plan of care to include primary care treatment, initial rehabilitation with projected goals, and projected timeframe of return to play needs to be addressed shortly after the incident of injury.

Many of the manual testing procedures for the shoulder have come under scrutiny recently. One study evaluating assessment of the impingement tests demonstrated the pooled sensitivity and specificity scores of the Neer test were 79% and 53%, respectively, and for the Hawkins-Kennedy test, the pooled sensitivity and specificity scores were 79% and 59%, respectively. These results led the authors to suggest that there is a lack of clarity regarding whether the special tests performed in a clinical evaluation are useful in differentially diagnosing shoulder pathologies.[6]

Another study demonstrated individual special test capabilities in determining superior labral anterior posterior (SLAP) lesion accuracy. Their finding through a decade of manuscripts demonstrated no single independent special test could be used as an accurate determining factor of a torn labrum.[7]

Technology has played a significant role in differential diagnosis regarding shoulder pathology. The use of magnetic resonance imaging (MRI),its diagnostic benefits, efficacy, and overutilization have been debated openly. Computed tomography (CT) and diagnostic ultrasound are also beneficial in many instances. The benefits of MRI can assist with the capsular laxity following shoulder dislocation,[8] while MRI arthrography appears to be the gold standard in diagnosing labral tears.[9–11]

Injuries associated with the shoulder can be classified as traumatic, overuse or biomechanical secondary to trauma or overuse or none of these.

TRAUMATIC
AC Sprain

AC sprains are classified by Rockwood[12] as

Type 1—minor sprain of AC ligament, intact joint capsule, intact coraco-clavicular (CC) ligament, intact deltoid and trapezius

Type 2—rupture of AC ligament and joint capsule, sprain of CC ligament but CC interspace intact, minimal detachment of deltoid and trapezius

Type 3—rupture of AC ligament, joint capsule, and CC ligament; clavicle elevated (as much as 100% displacement); detachment of deltoid and trapezius

Type 4—rupture of AC ligament, joint capsule, and CC ligament; clavicle displaced posteriorly into the trapezius; detachment of deltoid and trapezius

Type 5—rupture of AC ligament, joint capsule, and CC ligament; clavicle elevated (more than 100% displacement); detachment of deltoid and trapezius

Type 6 (rare)—rupture of AC ligament, joint capsule, and CC ligament; clavicle displaced behind the tendons of the biceps and coracobrachialis

Common mechanisms of injury to the AC joint include falling on an outstretched arm (FOOSH), or more frequently, direct trauma to the apex of the shoulder with the arm in adduction. Direct contact to the clavicle is more likely to present with a fractured clavicle than an AC separation, as the forces generated to fracture the clavicle are one sixth of those necessary to separate the AC joint.[12,13]

Patients commonly complain of superior shoulder pain increased with attempts of upper extremity elevation, with point tenderness at the AC joint. Weighted radiograph demonstrates the separation at the AC joint.

Treatment considerations are based upon the classification of severity. Type 1 and 2 sprains follow conservative treatment protocols including early intervention of cryotherapy, immobilization, and rest. Type 3 have come under scrutiny regarding surgical intervention, while types 4 through 6 usually require surgery.[14–16]

Key points to remember include
Properly diagnose the level of severity
Immobilization 2 to 4 weeks followed by physical therapy

Return-to-play criteria: painless motion, manual 5/5 strength on flexion and horizontal adduction/abduction, ability to perform shoulder press and bench press without pain

CLAVICLE FRACTURE

Clavicle fractures are common injuries, representing about 5% of emergency room fractures and 35% to 45% of all fractures that occur in the shoulder girdle area. The most frequent site of injury is at the middle third (group 1 fracture).[17] The most commonly used classification is the Allman scheme with the Neer modification as listed in **Box 1**.[18,19]

Common mechanisms of injury include falling directly on the shoulder (70%),[20] direct contact to the clavicle, or less commonly a FOOSH mechanism. Sports including football, soccer, martial arts, rugby, and wrestling may be associated with clavicle fractures.

Patients commonly will present with pain with upper extremity motion, with noted crepitus with any activity. The most frequent age group is youth through early 20s. Males are five times more frequent than females.[21] Although most present with a simple fracture, potential complications and underlying related traumatic conditions could exist, including brachial plexus and potential subclavian artery involvement.[22,23]

Initial treatment includes immobilization in a figure-8 splint for 2 to 4 weeks with re-evaluation to follow. Upon re-evaluation, ensuring proper shoulder mechanics could be reviewed, and 2 to 4 weeks of physical therapy could be indicated.

Key points to remember include
Proper classification of injury
Compliance is a concern in this population with this bracing
Return to play following 2 to 4 weeks immobilization, complete ROM of all facets of the shoulder complex, strength 5/5, particularly in flexion and ABD

Box 1
Allman scheme with Neer modification

Group 1—fracture of middle third

Group 2—fracture of the distal third

    Type 1—minimally displaced/interligamentous

    Type 2—displaced because of fracture medial to the coracoclavicular ligaments

        2A—both the conoid and trapezoid remain attached to distal fragment

        2B—either the conoid is torn or both the conoid and trapezoid are torn

    Type 3—fractures involving articular surface

    Type 4—ligaments intact to the periosteum with displacement of the proximal fragment

    Type 5—comminuted

Group 3—fracture of the proximal third

    Type 1—minimal displacement

    Type 2—displaced

    Type 3—intra-articular

    Type 4—epiphyseal separation (observed in patients aged 25 years and younger)

    Type 5—comminuted

DISLOCATED SHOULDER

The shoulder is the most frequently dislocated joint in the body.[24] Because of the vast mobility required for athletic activity, the ligaments and muscles that stabilize the glenohumeral joint are under constant challenge. Dislocations that occur in the teenage years have a greater than 70% chance of reoccurring. Anterior dislocations occur in approximately 95% of the instances, with posterior and inferior dislocations encompassing the latter 5%.[25]

Mechanism of injury most frequently associated with anterior dislocation includes simultaneous humeral abduction, external rotation against a force of external rotation, and horizontal extension. Common sports mechanisms include football arm tackling, baseball sliding, and wrestling switching. Additionally, less common positions included forward falling creating a hyperflexion/external rotation glenohumeral position.

On-the-field presentation commonly includes complaints of pain with the joint in a stuck position, where anatomically the humeral head is caught on the rim of the glenoid, with surrounding muscular in constant contraction attempting self-reduction. Once reduction has been completed, radiographs are imperative. Clinically, it is wiser to attain pre- and postreduction radiographs. Up to 72 hours after reduction, the athlete will demonstrate weakness in shoulder elevation and external rotation, with a positive apprehension sign. Additionally, associated damage including rotator cuff tear and brachial plexus involvement (shoulder unhappy triad)[26,27] and a common Bankart lesion with traumatic dislocations will be seen.

Initial treatment once was agreed upon by the medical community to consist of 4 to 6 weeks immobilization following the first dislocation, followed by a similar timeframe of rehabilitation. This continues to have support.[28] Numerous research, however, has demonstrated that a more considerable and immediate surgical repair is indicated for the young, active population sustaining an initial glenohumeral dislocation.[29–31] Extensive postsurgical rehabilitation is recommended.

Posterior dislocations commonly occur with a direct humeral head force while the arm is flexed, adducted, and internally rotated. Sports most commonly involved are football and lacrosse. The athlete may not directly recall an incident of injury; however, when placed in the previously referenced position, posterior discomfort is reproduced. Symptoms also are inferred with posterior capsule and ligamentous laxity, namely the coracohumeral and superior glenohumeral ligaments[32] and boney deformities that include increased humeral retroversion, glenoid retroversion, and glenoid hypoplasia.[33–35] Reverse Bankart lesions commonly are seen in these dislocations. One researcher found 100% of his 27 patients to have at least one lesion in the posterior–inferior labrum with a posterior dislocation.[36] Most posterior dislocations require surgical intervention because of these related anatomic conditions.

Key points to remember include
- On-the-field reduction is not recommended
- Always x-ray after reduction
- High incidence of Hill Sachs lesion (>70%) in first-time dislocation
- Sling and swathe for initial first 72 hours, pain control and cryotherapy
- Education in avoiding the abduction/external rotation position following dislocation, specifically while sleeping
- Many secondary and tertiary dislocations occur within the first week because of noncompliance issues

Strongly recommend orthopedic consult after initial dislocation.

Return to play following restored ROM, strength of 5/5 in abduction, internal and external rotation and flexion—must be able to protect the shoulder from position of injury mechanism

ROTATOR CUFF

The rotator cuff acts as the dynamic stabilizer, maintaining an instant center of motion between the head of the humerus and the glenoid.[37] When working efficiently, the larger muscles including the deltoid and latissimus dorsi can move the upper extremity with little movement away from the instant center of motion. Failure of the dynamic stabilizers will create undue stress at various anatomic areas, including the subacromion space, the deltoid insertion, and the biceps origin, as well as increase capsular stress, yielding increased shoulder laxity. This cycle will continue, adding stress to the rotator cuff muscles, eventually developing tendinitis and ultimate breakdown of the rotator cuff.

Overhead athletes are most susceptible to rotator cuff pathology, including tendinitis and tears. The mechanics of throwing or swinging a racquet overhead challenges the dynamic stabilizers in multiple ranges of motion. Athletes who demonstrate early fatigue of the rotator cuff develop compensatory movement patterns, exacerbating the mechanical quandary, by elevating the scapula to achieve the ultimate motion to allow for superior humeral translation.[38]

Most rotator cuff tears are associated with multiple microtrauma as previously outlined. Most of the degeneration occurs at the coracoacromial arch, which is comprised of the acromion, the coracoacromial ligament and the coracoid. The supraspinatus tendon runs through the arch. Changes in mechanics caused by fatigue (overuse), related injury or increased level of competition play a role in the mechanism. An emerging consensus suggests that the etiology of rotator cuff disease is multifactorial.[39]

The athlete will present with complaints of pain with activity and rest. Pain usually will be specific to the top of the shoulder ranging down along the mid-deltoid. Point tenderness may be noted in the greater tuberosity, the deltoid insertion, or the biceps tendon. ROM deficits and weakness will be associated with the symptoms. A history of specific traumatic incident, general shoulder pain, or previous tendinopathies will be presented. Generally, the functional inability to achieve the velocity, distance, or accuracy of a throw, serve or toss is the main reason medical intervention is sought. Any sport where there is overhead activity, throwing, repetitive motion, or long-term overhead positioning is included in this sequence of events.

Initial treatment of a suspected rotator cuff tear includes immobilization, cryotherapy, and MRI for further assessment. Surgical intervention is imminent for return to athletic activity.

Key points to remember include

Traumatic rotator cuff tears are associated with violent dislocations and related trauma. Extensive physical therapy using return of normal shoulder biomechanics, normal ROM, outlining high repetition, low resistance exercise protocols, and specific sport-related conditioning

Return to play depends upon many factors including upon the age of the patient, the severity of the pathology, the type of treatment rendered, and the expectations of the patient.

Type 2 acromion and type 3 acromion are common associated factors of rotator cuff tears[40,41]

SLAP LESION

The glenoid labrum surrounds the entire circumference of the glenoid surface.[42] Superiorly, the labrum is contiguous, with the tendon insertion of the long head of the biceps as it attaches to the supraglenoid tubercle. The glenoid labrum increases the area and depth of the glenoid cavity, contributing to articular stability of the glenohumeral joint. The labrum stabilizes the humeral head as it attempts to translate anteriorly or posteriorly upon the glenoid surface.[43] Biomechanically, the two structures most relevant to the stability of the labrum are the inferior glenohumeral ligament and the long head of the biceps.[44]

SLAP lesions have a distinctive classification, much as other shoulder injuries. In multiple studies, type 2 was most common.[45–47] They have been classified as follows[48]

Type 1—the glenoid labrum demonstrates degenerative changes and fraying at the edges but remains firmly attached to the glenoid rim; no avulsion of the biceps tendon is present.

Type 2—degenerative changes and fraying are present; the glenoid labrum is detached completely from the anterosuperior to the posterosuperior glenoid rim. This portion of the labrum is lifted by the long biceps tendon, and the attachment of the biceps tendon is unstable.

Type 3—the free margin of the superior labrum is displaced into the joint (bucket handle), whereas the labral attachment to the glenoid rim and biceps tendon remains intact. The insertion of the biceps tendon is not unstable.

Type 4—the superior portion of the labrum is displaced into the joint (bucket handle); in contrast to type 3 tears, the long biceps tendon also is affected, involving partial rupture in the direction of the fibers.

Most SLAP lesions occur in conjunction with other shoulder disorders, making the mechanism of injury and the diagnosis difficult to establish. Traumatic occurrences include high-speed falls, in skiing or wakeboarding, while others will include direct trauma. In sports medicine, however, the most common is the overhead, repetitive athlete, where the labrum may be a single traumatic throw, or a result of repetitive microtrauma.

The athlete will present with deep joint pain specific to glenohumeral ROM associated with sport-specific activity. Most common are the pain within the arc of motion, weakness, and decreases in functional ROM, depending upon location and structures torn.

Because of the propensity of multiple structures of involvement, initial treatment includes immobilization and addressing of symptomatic complaints while instituting specific imaging studies to differentiate structures. MRI arthrography is the gold standard for diagnosing labral tears.[11]

Key points to remember include

Regimented physical therapy should follow surgery immediately for up to 4 to 6 months.

When previous conservative therapy for biceps tendinitis that has failed to restore function, one should consider labral involvement.

Young adolescent throwers are more common for tendinitis, while physically developed high school and college throwers will shear the labrum.

OVERUSE AND BIOMECHANICAL
Biceps Tendinitis

The anatomic position and function of the long head of the biceps tendon lends itself to primary and secondary involvement of sports-related injury. The long head biceps tendon lies in the bicipital groove of the humerus between the greater and lesser tuberosities and angles 90° inward at the upper end of the groove, crossing the humeral head to insert at the upper edge of the glenoid labrum and supraglenoid tubercle.[49] It acts as a primary mover for forearm supination and elbow flexion. The tendon is a stabilizing force for the humerus during shoulder external rotation and abduction, a position most common in throwing.[50]

The mechanism of injury regarding an isolated biceps tendinitis is most common in overhead athletes, including baseball, javelin, tennis, lacrosse, and swimming, and repetitive bicep athletes such as weightlifters, wrestlers, and rowers.[51,52] Overutilization and mechanical changes caused by fatigue predispose this group. Direct trauma to the biceps is observed most commonly in high-repetition contact sports.

Multiple structure mechanisms, where the biceps tendinitis is associated include impingement, rotator cuff, SLAP lesions, and shoulder dislocation. Although bicipital tendinitis may be of lesser concern, its failure to be addressed will create havoc upon the rehabilitative goals of related trauma.

The athlete commonly will complain of functional pain and increased intensity at night and with activity, specifically overhead repetitive motion. Strength training also can increase symptoms. Point tenderness over the long head proximally and muscle tests regarding elbow flexion and Yergason and speed tests will be positive.

Initial care of removing the cause, nonsteroidal anti-inflammatory drugs (NSAIDs), and physical therapy modalities will decrease the symptoms. This, however, may not reduce reoccurrence if mechanics are the cause. In these athletic populations, it is the cause that must be addressed with greater concern than the associated symptoms. Chronicity regarding tendinitis will result in poor outcomes and unsatisfied patients.

Key points to remember include
Biceps tendinitis usually associated with mechanical dysfunction or overuse
Observed frequently in youth superstars, where they are pitching for multiple teams during a single timeframe
Increased levels of competition can be a causative factor
Iontophoresis is a common modality of choice
Rule out related mechanical diagnoses, including SLAP, impingement, and rotator cuff tendinitis
Return to play after symptoms are removed completely, and mechanical analysis has been determined

IMPINGEMENT SYNDROME

Neer[53] was the first to recognize the mechanical impingement of the rotator cuff within the coracoacromial arch. He further described three stages of impingement classification:

Stage 1, commonly affecting patients younger than 25 years, is depicted by acute inflammation, edema, and hemorrhage in the rotator cuff. This stage usually is reversible with nonoperative treatment.
Stage 2 usually affects patients aged 25 to 40 years, resulting as a continuum of stage 1. The rotator cuff tendon progresses to fibrosis and tendonitis, which commonly does not respond to conservative treatment and requires operative intervention.
Stage 3 commonly affects patients older than 40 years. As this condition progresses, it may lead to mechanical disruption of the rotator cuff tendon and to

changes in the coracoacromial arch with osteophytosis along the anterior acromion. Surgical I anterior acromioplasty and rotator cuff repair commonly are required.

Primary impingement often is considered due to overuse history of repetitive motion of overhead activity and fatigue, which alter normal shoulder mechanics.[54] Additionally associated are anatomically deviations of the acromion. Type 1 is flat (17%); type 2 is curved (43%), and type 3 is hooked (40%). The hooked configuration has been associated most strongly with full-thickness rotator cuff tears.[55]

Secondary impingement is associated with various related mechanical dysfunctions, muscular imbalances, or previous medical conditions. These conditions alter normal biomechanics, leading to structural changes on the rotator cuff tendons. These conditions must be addressed for a positive outcome to occur.

The athlete will present with progressive symptoms aggravated with overhead activity. General tenderness is found in the shoulder region during muscle testing, while point tenderness is noted at the greater tuberosity. Weakness on flexion, abduction, and external rotation also will be noticed. Neer and Empty Can tests will be positive.

Initial treatment should follow that of typical tendinitis, including ceasing activity, NSAIDs, and physical therapy modalities. Progressive exercise should follow the acute phase.

Key points to remember include
- Rule out differential diagnoses that will predispose impingement syndrome (SLAP, rotator cuff tear, multi-directional instability [MDI])
- Chronic complications could include calcifying tendinitis, although not commonly observed in the young population
- Educating the coach, parent, and athlete regarding mechanics and overuse
- Perform a mechanical evaluation focused on the cause rather than the symptoms
- Return to play when symptoms have subsided and cause is addressed

ADHESIVE CAPSULITIS

Adhesive capsulitis, or frozen shoulder syndrome, is the reduction of passive and active ROM of the glenohumeral and periscapular motions of the shoulder. Symptoms may be isolated with insidious onset, or related to other pathologies, including fractured humerus, rotator cuff, impingement, or any required immobilized time period.

Lundberg divided the two different causes into primary and secondary groups.[56] Criteria were established for both groups to include painful shoulder with limitation in both active and passive ranges of motion lasting at least 1 month in both glenohumeral and scapulothoracic joints. Furthermore, patients had to determine if the pain and limitations had plateaued or increased. Symptoms that improved did not meet the criteria. Primary symptoms included insidious onset, gradual loss of motion, increased functional stiffness, and ultimately mild improvement. The secondary group was differentiated from the primary by including a definitive mechanism, suggesting related pathology.

Sports medicine usually includes the secondary group, where a mechanical change took place through trauma, or immobilization in the attempt to allow the glenohumeral joint to settle down, after a fracture or surgery. This group includes athletes complaining of lost ROM, weakness, and general dysfunction. Because of multiple attempts to elevate the arm using compensatory musculature following immobilization, the athlete may complain of upper trapezius, cervical, and deltoid pain.

Initial treatment in the athletic population includes avoidance of prolonged immobilization with related pathologies if possible, including conservative overuse of a sling. Once cleared to resume activity, immediate physical therapy is indicated to improve the normal kinematics at both the glenohumeral and the scapulothoracic joints.

Key points to remember include
Home programs are usually ineffective with this syndrome.
Diabetics have a significantly higher incidence of frozen shoulder than the nondiabetic population.
Manipulation under anesthesia should be a final effort to attain mild-to-moderate improvement in functional motion.
Aggressive rehabilitation must be used in severe cases of adhesive capsulitis; however, one must consider the related pathologies associated with the condition and the contraindications.
Flexion, abduction, and internal and external rotation are affected by the adhesion of the inferior pouch, causing moderate-to-severe limitation in the athletic population.Return to play once normal kinematics, strength, and ROM have been restored; less than that, related pathologies will arise.

MDI

MDI first was diagnosed in 1980 by Neer and Foster.[57] Essentially, the capsular ligaments have been stretched, reducing their capacity to maintain static stability within the glenohumeral joint, allowing for multiplanar laxity throughout the joint.[58]

Hawkins[59] and others established criteria using two mnemonic devices, concerning shoulder instability. They are TUBS and AMBRII; AMBRII is used for multidirectional instabilities (**Box 2**).

MDI is not a sport or positional-related diagnosis; however, it commonly is observed in populations of gymnasts and swimmers. Athletes will present with general bilateral shoulder soreness and inflammation, either sports activity-related, or positional related as in sleeping. Insidious onset is the norm, and variable structures of pain may lead one to initially consider the patient a symptom magnifier. Related pathologies including biceps tendinitis, impingement syndrome, and dislocation and subluxation are common.[60]

Upon evaluation, there is a positive sulcus sign bilaterally, with poor capsular end feel during passive range of motion evaluation. Often the youth athlete is not considered to have MDI because of the normal hyperlaxity expected at the age. These symptoms do not diminish with maturity. Generally, imaging studies are inconclusive. False-positive special tests are not uncommon; however, instability is greater than complaints of reproducible pain.

Initial treatment is long-term physical therapy stabilization exercise regimens, up to 3 to 6 months. Compliance and direction are imperative, suggesting that a program associated with a typical fitness gym membership will fall short of expected goals. Initiation of scapulothoracic stability and the larger muscle groups surrounding the shoulder complex is essential. Early rehabilitative complaints may increase if there is no scapulothoracic stabilization, leading to increased inflammation of the glenohumeral joint.

Box 2
TUBS and AMBRII defined

TUBS

    T raumatic etiology

    U nidirectional instability

    B ankart lesion

    S urgical repair

AMBRII

    A traumatic etiology

    M ultidirectional instability

    B ilateral involvement

    R ehabilitative initial management

    Rotator Interval tightening with Inferior capsular shift repairs

---

Key points to remember include

    Recognition of AMBRII patient presentation—bilateral is key sign

    Removing activity that is causing symptoms

    Specific exercise protocol designed to stabilize by strengthening stabilizers before progressing to typical machine exercises

    Exercise compliance issues in this population

    Orthopedic consult if rehabilitation fails

    Return to activity with gradual addition of components of sport without increased symptoms—may require a season off

SUMMARY

The shoulder complex remains one of the more challenging areas to ascertain complete comprehension of all of the intricacies involved because of its many moving parts and the relationships they have upon each joint. Each evaluation must take into account the effects the involved joint has upon the other three with respect to biomechanics of a multi-joint process. Much like a billiard player, each decision must be made with a thorough understanding as to the net effects that decision will have upon each joint within the complex. Simply addressing the involved joint may create additional mechanical challenges, thereby creating yet another problem.

There are no single easy answers to evaluating the shoulder and developing a plan of care. There is no single special test, single imaging study, or single question to simplify the process. Developing an appreciation of the complexity that allows normal human movement of the upper extremity requires clinicians to be thorough.

REFERENCES

1. Perry J. Normal upper extremity kinesiology. Phys Ther 1978;58:265.
2. Ludewig PM, Phadke V, Braman JP, et al. Motion of shoulder complex during multiplanar humeral elevation. J Bone Joint Surg Am 2009;91(2):378–89.
3. Enoka RM, Duchateau J. Muscle fatigue: what, why and how it influences muscle function. J Physiol 2008;586:11–23.

4. Akel I, Pekmezci M, Hayran M, et al. Evaluation of shoulder balance in the normal adolescent population and its correlation with radiological parameters. Eur Spine J 2008;17(3):348–54.

5. Oyama S, Myers JB, Wassinger CA, et al. Asymmetric resting scapular posture in healthy overhead athletes. J Athl Train 2008;43(6):565–70.

6. Hegedus EJ, Goode A, Campbell S, et al. Physical examination tests of the shoulder: a systematic review with meta-analysis of individual tests. Br J Sports Med 2008;42(2):80–92.

7. Dessaur WA, Magarev ME. Diagnostic accuracy of clinical tests for superior labral anterior posterior lesions: a systemic review. J Orthop Sports Phys Ther 2008; 38(6):341–52.

8. Ng AW, Chu CM, Lo WN, et al. Assessment of capsular laxity with recurrent anterior dislocation using MRI. AJR Am J Roentgenol 2009;192(6):1690–5.

9. Magee T. 3-T MRI of the shoulder: is MR arthrography necessary? Am J Roentgenol 2009;192(1):86–92.

10. Woertler K, Waldt S. MRI imaging in sports-related glenohumeral instability. Eur Radiol 2006;16(12):2622–36.

11. Waldt S, Burkart A, Lange P, et al. Diagnostic performance of MR arthrography in the assessment of superior labral anteroposterior lesions of the shoulder. AJR Am J Roentgenol 2004;182:1271–8.

12. Rockwood CA, Green DP, editors. Injuries to the acromioclavicular joint. Fractures in adults. Philadelphia: JB Lippincott; 1984. p. 860–91.

13. Macdonald PB, Lapointe P. Acromioclavicular and sternoclavicular joint injuries. Orthop Clin North Am 2008;39(4):535–45.

14. Choi SW, Lee TJ, Moon KH, et al. Minimally invasive coracoclavicular stabilization with suture anchors for acute acromioclavicular dislocation. Am J Sports Med 2008;36(5):961–5.

15. Rolf O, Hann von Weyhern A, Ewers A, et al. Acromioclavicular dislocation Rockwood III-V: results of early versus delayed surgical treatment. Arch Orthop Trauma Surg 2007;128(10):1153–7.

16. Kumar S, Penematsa SR, Selvan T. Surgical reconstruction for chronic painful acromioclavicular joint dislocations. Arch Orthop Trauma Surg 2007;127(6):481–4.

17. Rubino LJ, Lawless MW. Clavicle fractures. Available at: http://emedicine.medscape.com/article/1260953-overview.

18. Allman FL. Fractures and ligamentous injuries of the clavicle and its articulation. J Bone Joint Surg Am 1967;49(4):774–84.

19. Neer CS 2nd. Fractures of the distal third of the clavicle. Clin Orthop 1968;58:43–50.

20. Nowak J, Mallmin H, Larsson S. The aetiology and epidemiology of clavicular fractures. A prospective study during a two-year period in Uppsala, Sweden. Injury 2000;31(5):353–8.

21. White B, Epstein D, Sanders S, et al. Acute acromioclavicular injuries in adults. Orthopedics 2008;31(12):12.

22. Katras T, Baltazar U, Rush DS, et al. Subclavian arterial injury associated with blunt trauma. Vasc Surg 2001;35(1):43–50.

23. Kendall KM, Burton JH, Cushing B. Fatal subclavian artery transection from isolated clavicle fracture. J Trauma 2000;48(2):316–8.

24. Matsen FA III, Thomas SC, Rockwood CA Jr. Anterior glenohumeral instability. In: Rockwood CA Jr, Matsen FA III, editors, The shoulder, vol. 1. Philadelphia: WB Saunders Company; 1990. p. 526–622.

25. Dodson CC, Cordasco FA. Anterior glenohumeral joint dislocations. Orthop Clin North Am 2008;39(4):507–18.

26. Martin SS, Limbard TJ. The terrible triad of the shoulder. J South Orthop Assoc 1999;8(1):57–60.
27. Guven O, Akbar Z, Yalcin S, et al. Concomitant rotator cuff tear and brachial plexus injury in association with anterior shoulder dislocation:unhappy triad of the shoulder. J Orthop Trauma 1994;8(5):429–30.
28. Hovelius L, Olofsson A, Sandstrom B, et al. Nonoperative treatment of primary anterior shoulder dislocation in patients forty years of age and younger. A prospective twenty-five year follow-up. J Bone Joint Surg Am 2008;90(5):945–52.
29. Bedi A, Ryu RK. The treatment of primary anterior shoulder dislocations. Instr Course Lect 2009;58:293–304.
30. Robinson CM, Howes J, Murdoch H, et al. Functional outcome and risk of recurrent instability after primary traumatic anterior shoulder dislocation in young patients. J Bone Joint Surg Am 2006;88(11):2326–36.
31. Good CR, MacGillivray JD. Traumatic shoulder dislocation in the adolescent athlete:advances in surgical treatment. Curr Opin Pediatr 2005;17(1):25–9.
32. Pagnani MJ, Warren RF. Stabilizers of the glenohumeral joint. J Shoulder Elbow Surg 1994;3:173–90.
33. Wilson JC, McKeever FM. Traumatic posterior (retrograde) dislocation of the humerus. J Bone Joint Surg Am 1949;31:160–72.
34. Brewer BJ, Wubben RC, Carrera GF. Excessive retroversion of the glenoid cavity. A cause of nontraumatic posterior instability of the shoulder. J Bone Joint Surg Am 1986;68(5):724–31.
35. Hurley JA, Anderson TE, Dear W, et al. Posterior shoulder instability. Surgical versus conservative results with evaluation of glenoid version. Am J Sports Med 1992;20(4):396–400.
36. Kim SH, Ha KI, Park JS, et al. Arthroscopic posterior labral repair and capsular shift for traumatic unidirectional recurrent posterior subluxation of the shoulder. J Bone Joint Surg Am 2003;85(8):1479–87.
37. Wuelker N, Korell M, Thren K. Dynamic glenohumeral joint stability. J Shoulder Elbow Surg 1998;7(1):43–52.
38. Teyhen DS, Miller JM, Middag TR, et al. Rotator cuff fatigue and glenohumeral kinematics in participants without shoulder dysfunction. J Athl Train 2008;43(4):352–8.
39. Ecklund KJ, Lee TQ, Tibone J, et al. Rotator cuff tear arthropathy. J Am Acad Orthop Surg 2007;15(6):340–9.
40. Bigliani LU, Morrison DS, April EW. The morphology of the acromion and its relationship to rotator cuff tears. Orthop Trans 1986;10:228.
41. Yamanaka K, Fukda H. Aging process of the supraspinatus tendon in surgical disorders of the shoulder. In: Watson N, editor. Surgical disorders of the shoulder. New York: Churchill Livingstone; 1991. p. 247.
42. Moseley H, Overgaard B. The anterior capsular mechanism in recurrent anterior dislocation of the shoulder. Morphological and clinical studies with special reference to the glenoid labrum and glenohumeral ligaments. J Bone Joint Surg Br 1962;44B:913–27.
43. Turkel SJ, Panio MW, Marshall JL, et al. Stabilizing mechanisms preventing anterior dislocation of the glenohumeral joint. J Bone Joint Surg Am 1981;63(8):1208–17.
44. McGlynn FJ, Caspari RB. Arthroscopic findings in the subluxating shoulder. Clin Orthop Relat Res 1984;183:173–8.
45. Snyder SJ, Banas MP, Karzel RP. An analysis of 140 injuries to the superior glenoid labrum. J Shoulder Elbow Surg 1995;4(4):243–8.

46. Kim TK, Queale WS, Cosgarea AJ, et al. Clinical features of the different types of SLAP lesions: an analysis of one hundred and thirty-nine cases. J Bone Joint Surg Am 2003;85A:66–71.
47. Kampa RJ, Clasper J. Incidence of SLAP lesions in a military population. J R Army Med Corps 2005;151(3):171–5.
48. Snyder SJ, Karzel RP, Del Pizzo W, et al. SLAP lesions of the shoulder. Arthroscopy 1990;6(4):274–9.
49. Ahrens PM, Boileau P. The long head of biceps and associated tendinopathy. J Bone Joint Surg Br 2007;89(8):1001–9.
50. Nicholis JA, Hershman EB, editors. Bicipital tendinitis. The upper extremity in sports medicine. 2nd edition. St Louis (MO): Mosby; 1995. p. 303–6.
51. Ouellette H, Labis J, Bredella M, et al. Spectrum of shoulder injuries in the baseball pitcher. Skeletal Radiol 2008;37(6):491–8.
52. Patton WC, McCluskey GM 3rd. Biceps tendinitis and subluxation. Clin Sports Med 2001;20(3):505–29.
53. Neer CS 2nd. Anterior acromioplasty for the chronic impingement syndrome in the shoulder: a preliminary report. J Bone Joint Surg Am 1972;54(1):41–50.
54. Royer PJ, Kane EJ, Parks KE, et al. Fluoroscopic assessment of rotator cuff fatigue on glenohumeral arthrokinematics in shoulder impingement syndrome. J Shoulder Elbow Surg 2009 [Epub ahead of print].
55. DeBarardino TM, Chang WK. Shoulder impingement syndrome. Available at: http://emedicine.medscape.com/article/92974-overview.
56. Lundberg BJ. The frozen shoulder. Clinical and radiographical observations. The effect of manipulation under general anesthesia. Structure and glycosaminoglycan content of the joint capsule. Local bone metabolism. Acta Orthop Scand Suppl 1969;119:1–59.
57. Neer CS, Foster CR. Inferior capsular shift for involuntary inferior and multidirectional instability of the shoulder. A preliminary report. J Bone Joint Surg Am 1980; 62(6):897–908.
58. Castagna A, Nordenson U, Garofalo R, et al. Minor shoulder instability. Arthroscopy 2007;23(2):211–5.
59. Hawkins RJ, Bokor DJ. Clinical evaluation of shoulder problems. In: Rockwood CA, Matsen FA, editors. The shoulder. 2nd edition. Philadelphia: WB Saunders; 1990. p. 151.
60. Tibone JE, Elrod B, Jobe FW, et al. Surgical treatment of tears of the rotator cuff in athletes. J Bone Joint Surg Am 1986;68(6):887–91.

Rehabilitation of the Elbow Following Sports Injury

Todd S. Ellenbecker, DPT, MS, SCS, OCS, CSCS[a],*,
Tad E. Pieczynski, MS, PT, OCS, CSCS[a],
George J. Davies, DPT, MEd, SCS, ATC, CSCS[b]

KEYWORDS
- Elbow injury • Rehabilitation program
- Tendonitis • Tendonosis

Injuries to the elbow occur frequently in the overhead athlete due to the repetitive loads and forceful muscular activations inherent in throwing, hitting, serving, and spiking.[1,2] The most common injuries in the athlete include humeral epicondylitis, valgus extension overload, and ulnar collateral ligament injury.[3,4] The initial upper extremity evaluation including radiographs is the critical first step in early recognition and diagnosis of elbow injury, and allows for the referral to physical therapy whereby a comprehensive rehabilitation program can be initiated. The purpose of this article is to review the common elbow injuries in the overhead athlete and clinical tests used to confirm them, in addition to providing key concepts in the rehabilitation programs used to treat individuals with elbow injury and return them to high-level overhead activity.

COMMON INJURIES IN THE ATHLETE'S ELBOW

One of the most common overuse injuries of the elbow is humeral epicondylitis.[5,6] The repetitive overuse reported as one of the primary causative factors is particularly evident in the history of many athletic patients with elbow dysfunction. Epidemiologic research on adult tennis players reports incidences of humeral epicondylitis ranging from 35% to 50%.[7-11] This incidence is actually far greater than that reported in elite junior players (11%–12%) (United States Tennis Association, unpublished data, 1992).[12]

Reported in the literature as early as 1873 by Runge,[13] humeral epicondylitis or "tennis elbow" as it is more popularly known, has been extensively studied by many investigators. Cyriax,[14] in 1936, listed 26 causes of tennis elbow, and an extensive study of this overuse disorder by Goldie[15] in 1964 reported hypervascularization

[a] Physiotherapy Associates Scottsdale Sports Clinic, 9917 North 95th Street, Scottsdale, AZ 85258, USA
[b] Armstrong Atlantic State University, Savannah, GA, USA
* Corresponding author.
E-mail address: ellenbeckerpt@cox.net (T.S. Ellenbecker).

of the extensor aponeurosis and an increased quantity of free nerve endings in the subtendinous space. Leadbetter[16] described humeral epicondylitis as a degenerative condition consisting of a time-dependent process including vascular, chemical, and cellular events that lead to a failure of the cell-matrix healing response in human tendon. This description of tendon injury differs from earlier theories in which an inflammatory response was considered as a primary factor, hence the term "tendonitis" was used as opposed to the term recommended by Leadbetter[16] and Nirschl.[17]

Nirschl[4,6,17] and Nirschl and Ashman[18] have defined humeral epicondylitis as an extra-articular tendonous injury characterized by excessive vascular granulation and an impaired healing response in the tendon, which they have termed "angiofibroblastic hyperplasia." In a thorough histopathological analysis, Nirschl and colleagues[19] studied specimens of injured tendon obtained from areas of chronic overuse and reported that they do not contain large numbers of lymphocytes, macrophages, and neutrophils. Instead, tendonosis seems to be a degenerative process characterized by large populations of fibroblasts, disorganized collagen, and vascular hyperplasia.[19] It is not clear why tendonosis is painful, given the lack of inflammatory cells, and it is also unknown why the collagen does not mature. Nirschl[17] has described the primary structure involved in lateral humeral epicondylitis as the tendon of the extensor carpi radialis brevis. Approximately one-third of cases involve the tendon of the extensor communis.[19] In addition, the extensor carpi radialis longus and extensor carpi ulnaris can be involved. The primary site of medial humeral epicondylitis is the flexor carpi radialis, pronator teres, and flexor carpi ulnaris tendons.[6,17] Finally, Nirschl[17] reports that the incidence of lateral humeral epicondylitis is far greater than that of medial epicondylitis in recreational tennis players and in the leading arm (left arm in a right-handed golfer), whereas medial humeral epicondylitis is far more common in elite tennis players and throwing athletes, due to the powerful loading of the flexor and pronator muscle tendon units during the valgus extension overload inherent in the acceleration phase of those overhead movement patterns. In addition, the trailing arm of the golfer (right arm in a right-handed golfer) is reportedly more likely to have medial symptoms than lateral.

Repeated activities such as overhead throwing, tennis serving, or throwing the javelin can lead to characteristic patterns of osseous and osteochondral injury in the older active patient as well as the adolescent elbow. These injuries are commonly referred to as valgus extension overload injuries (Fig. 1).[20] As a result of the valgus stress incurred during throwing or the serving motion, traction placed via the medial aspect of the elbow can create body spurs or osteophytes at the medial epicondyle or coronoid process of the elbow.[21–23] In addition, the valgus stress during elbow extension creates impingement, which leads to the development of osteophyte formation at the posterior and posteriomedial aspects of the olecranon tip, causing chondromalacia and loose body formation.[20] The combined motion of valgus pressure with the powerful extension of the elbow leads to posterior osteophyte formation, due to impingement of the posterior medial aspect of the ulna against the trochlea and olecranon fossa. Joyce and colleagues[24] have reported the presence of chondromalacia in the medial groove of the trochlea, which often precedes osteophyte formation. Erosion to subchondral bone is often witnessed when olecranon osteophytes are initially developing. Injury to the ulnar collateral ligament and medial muscle tendon units of the flexor-pronator group can also occur with this type of repetitive loading.[22,25]

During the valgus stress that occurs to the human elbow during the acceleration phase of both the throwing and serving motions, lateral compressive forces occur in the lateral aspect of the elbow, specifically at the radiocapitellar joint. Of great concern

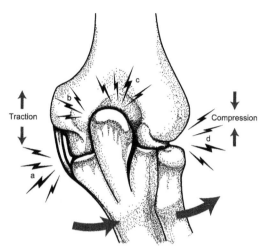

Fig. 1. Osteochondral injury from valgus extension overload mechanism of the overhead throwing motion.

in the immature pediatric throwing athlete is osteochondritis dissecans (OCD) and Panner disease.[3,24] Although the incidence of OCD and Panner disease is low, the importance of obtaining radiographs in the thorough evaluation of the pediatric elbow cannot be understated. The presence of OCD and Panner disease, though not common, should be ruled out in every case.[26] The characteristics of Panner disease are for the presence of fissuring and increased density of the captiellum.[26] The most common onset age of both Panner disease and OCD is less than 10 years, occurring most commonly in males, and typically in the dominant arm.[27] In the older adult elbow, the radiocapitellar joint can be the site of joint degeneration and osteochondral injury from the compressive loading.[22] This lateral compressive loading is increased in the elbow, with medial ulnar collateral ligament laxity or ligament injury.[3]

SPECIAL CONSIDERATIONS FOR THE ADOLESCENT ATHLETE'S ELBOW

Injuries to the throwing arm in the adolescent athlete occur frequently due to the highly repetitive nature of baseball, tennis, and other overhead sports. The increased demands of early sport specialization and year-round participation required to obtain success and develop high levels of skill in these overhead sports can subject the adolescent's shoulder and elbow to injury. A recent epidemiologic report studying youth sport participation and injury risk concluded that participation in several sports (multiple) seemed to have a protective effect from the harmful risks of single-sport participation.[28] Despite these findings, clinicians frequently find extensive single-sport participation histories when evaluating young athletes with shoulder and elbow injury. This high participation can lead to extensive musculoskeletal adaptation and eventual injury. One of the primary unique concerns for any clinician working with the adolescent thrower with shoulder or elbow pain of overuse origin is the growth plate (**Fig. 2**). Knowledge of anatomic and developmental factors inherent in the adolescent's upper extremity can guide clinicians during evaluation and treatment of overuse injuries. Repetitive valgus extension stresses applied to the young overhead athlete can lead to injury of the apophyseal growth plate (physes) in the elbow. Acute injury to the medial epicondylar apophysis can be in the form of an avulsion, with chronic

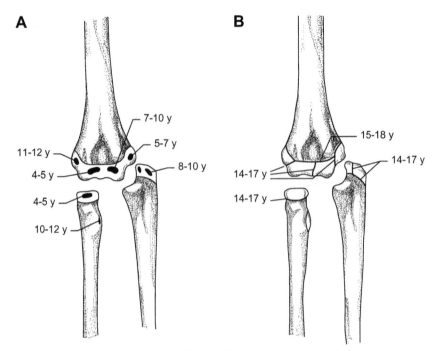

Fig. 2. Growth plates of the human elbow with approximate time of closure.

stress leading to traction apophysitis. Apophyseal separation will occur in adolescents, instead of rupture of the ulnar collateral ligament.[24] The cartilaginous growth plate represents the weak link, and before fusion of the secondary ossification center, strong forceful contraction of the flexor pronator musculature that occurs during the acceleration phase of the throwing motion or overhead serving motion in tennis can cause apophyseal separation. The growth plate is a cartilaginous disc between the apophysis and metaphysis of the bone. The site of separation of the growth plate is frequently between the calcified and uncalcified cartilage matrix. The relatively small amount of calcified matrix at this level accounts for the relative weakness of the growth plate, making the area vulnerable to injury with repeated stresses, particularly during the valgus stress coupled with extension at the elbow with overhead throwing.

Ossification centers of primary importance to the overhead throwing athlete are the medial epicondyle and olecranon ossification centers. The medial epicondyle ossification center is the second ossification center to appear at age 4 and develops slowly, and is the last center to unite with the humeral shaft, as late as 15 to 16 years of age.[29] The olecranon ossification center usually develops at approximately 9 years of age and begins to unite at age 14. The high-intensity muscular contraction of the triceps, through its insertion on the olecranon during the acceleration of throwing and serving motions, may create problems in this important region. These osseous injuries further support standard radiography of the elbow during the comprehensive evaluation process, before commencement of a rehabilitation program. Additional ossification centers (with the date of appearance) include the capitellum (2 years), radial head (4 years), medial epicondyle (4 years), trochlea (7 years), olecranon (9 years), and lateral epicondyle (10 years). Because the soft tissue surrounding the apophyses is stronger than the cartilage present at the apophyses, injurious forces causing a sprain or strain in an adult may cause an avulsion fracture in children.[24] The most common site for an avulsion fracture is the medial epicondyle. The avulsion commonly occurs during the late cocking/early acceleration phase of throwing, when a pop may be heard at the time of injury. The Salter-Harris classification system[30] is commonly used to describe acute physeal injuries. The reader is referred to this reference for a more complete discussion of this important classification.

CLINICAL EXAMINATION OF THE ELBOW

Structural inspection of the patient's elbow must include a complete and thorough inspection of the entire upper extremity and trunk.[3] The heavy reliance on the kinetic chain for power generation and the important role of the elbow as a link in the kinetic chain necessitates the examination of the entire upper extremity and trunk in the clinical evaluation.[3,31] However, because many overuse injuries occur in athletic individuals, structural inspection of the patient or athlete with an injured elbow can be complicated by a lack of bilateral symmetry in the upper extremities. Adaptive changes are commonly encountered during clinical examination of the athletic elbow, particularly in the unilaterally dominant upper extremity athlete. In these athletes, use of the contralateral extremity as a baseline is particularly important to determine the degree of actual adaptation that may be a contributing factor in the patient's injury presentation. A brief overview of the common adaptations that have been reported in the literature can provide valuable information to assist the clinician during the structural inspection of the injured athlete with elbow pain.

Several classic studies have reported on elbow range of motion adaptations. King and colleagues[32] initially reported on elbow range of motion in professional baseball pitchers. Fifty percent of the pitchers examined were found to have a flexion contracture of the dominant elbow, with 30% of subjects demonstrating a cubitus valgus deformity. Chinn and colleagues[33] measured world-class professional adult tennis players and reported significant elbow flexion contractures on the dominant arm as well. More recently, Ellenbecker and colleagues[34] measured elbow flexion contractures averaging 5° in a population of 40 healthy professional baseball pitchers. Directly related to elbow function was wrist flexibility, which Ellenbecker and colleagues[34] reported as significantly less in extension on the dominant arm due to tightness of the wrist flexor musculature, with no difference in wrist flexion range of motion between extremities. Wright and colleagues[35] reported on 33 throwing athletes before the competitive season. The average loss of elbow extension was 7° and the average loss of flexion was 5.5°. Ellenbecker and Roetert (Ellenbecker TS, Roetert EP, unpublished data, 1994) measured senior tennis players aged 55 years and older, and found flexion contractures averaging 10° in the dominant elbow as well as significantly less wrist flexion range of motion. The higher use of the wrist extensor musculature is likely the cause of limited wrist flexor range of motion among the senior tennis players, as opposed to the reduced wrist extension range of motion from excessive overuse of the wrist flexor muscles inherent in baseball pitching.[2,36]

Although it is beyond the scope of this article, it is imperative that glenohumeral joint rotational range of motion be measured due to the important role of glenohumeral internal rotation deficiency in valgus loading of the throwing elbow.[37] For a complete discussion of glenohumeral joint rotational measurement with scapular stabilization, the reader is referred to these references.[38–41] Identification of a loss of glenohumeral joint internal rotation and, more importantly, loss of total rotation range of motion with internal rotation range of motion loss would lead the clinician to interventions to address the proximal rotational deficiency in addition to providing proximal stabilization of the scapulothoracic and glenohumeral joints.

In summary, based on the findings of these descriptive profiles, the finding of an elbow flexion contracture and limited wrist flexion or extension range of motion, as well as reduced glenohumeral joint internal rotation, can be expected during the examination of an athlete from a unilaterally dominant upper extremity sport. Careful measurement during the clinical examination is recommended to determine baseline levels of range of motion loss in the distal upper extremity.

Several studies have also been published regarding osseous adaptations in the athletic elbow. In a study by Priest and colleagues,[42] 84 world-ranked tennis players were studied using radiography, and an average of 6.5 bony changes were found on the dominant elbow of each player. In addition, Priest and colleagues reported 2 times as many bony adaptations, such as spurs, on the medial aspect of the elbow compared with the lateral aspect. The coronoid process of the ulna was the number 1 site of osseous adaptation or spurring. An average 44% increase in thickness of the anterior humeral cortex was found on the dominant arm of these players, with an 11% increase in cortical thickness reported in the radius of the dominant tennis-playing extremity. In a magnetic resonance imaging (MRI) study, Waslewski and colleagues[43] found osteophytes at the proximal or distal insertion of the ulnar collateral ligament in 5 of 20 asymptomatic professional baseball pitchers, as well as posterior osteophytes in 2 of 20 pitchers.

Manual clinical examination of the human elbow to assess medial and lateral laxity can be challenging, given the presence of humeral rotation and small increases in joint opening that often present with ulnar collateral ligament injury. Ellenbecker and colleagues[34] measured medial elbow joint laxity in 40 asymptomatic professional baseball pitchers, to determine whether bilateral differences in medial elbow laxity exist in healthy pitchers with a long history of repetitive overuse to the medial aspect of the elbow. A Telos stress radiography device was used to assess medial elbow joint opening, using a standardized valgus stress of 15 daN (kilo-Pascals) with the elbow placed in 25° of elbow flexion and the forearm in a supinated position. The joint space between the medial epicondyle and coronoid process of the ulna was measured using anterior-posterior radiographs by a musculoskeletal radiologist and compared bilaterally, with and without the application of the valgus stress. Results showed significant differences between extremities with stress application, with the dominant elbow opening 1.20 mm and the nondominant elbow opening 0.88 mm. This difference, although statistically significant, averaged 0.32 mm between the dominant and nondominant elbow and would be virtually unidentifiable with manual assessment. Previous research by Rijke and colleagues[44] using stress radiography had identified a critical level of 0.5 mm increase in medial elbow joint opening in elbows with ulnar collateral ligament injury. Thus, the results of the study by Ellenbecker and colleagues[34] do support this 0.5-mm critical level, as asymptomatic professional pitchers in their study exhibited less than this 0.5 mm of medial elbow joint laxity.

In addition to the range of motion and osseous adaptations, muscular adaptations occur. Isometric grip strength measured using a hand grip dynamometer has revealed unilateral increases in strength in elite junior, adult, and senior tennis players ranging from 10% to 30% using standardized measurement methods.[3,33,45,46] Isokinetic dynamometers have been used to measure specific muscular performance parameters in elite-level tennis players and baseball pitchers.[3,45,47,48]

Ellenbecker[45] measured isokinetic wrist and forearm strength in mature adult tennis players who were highly skilled, and found 10% to 25% greater wrist flexion and extension as well as forearm pronation strength on the dominant extremity compared with the nondominant extremity. In addition, no significant difference between extremities in forearm supination strength was measured. No significant difference between extremities was found in elbow flexion strength in elite tennis players, but dominant arm elbow extension strength was significantly stronger than the non–tennis-playing extremity.[47] Research on professional throwing athletes has identified significantly greater wrist flexion and forearm pronation strength on the dominant arm by as much as 15% to 35% compared with the nondominant extremity,[3] with no difference in wrist extension strength or forearm supination strength between extremities. Wilk and colleagues[49] reported 10% to 20% greater elbow flexion strength in professional baseball pitchers on the dominant arm, as well as 5% to 15% greater elbow extension strength compared with the nondominant extremity.

These data help to portray the chronic muscular adaptations that can be present in the overhead athlete who may present with an elbow injury, as well as to determine realistic and accurate discharge strength levels following rehabilitation. Failure to return the stabilizing musculature to its often dominant status (10% to as much as 35%) on the dominant extremity in these athletes may represent an incomplete rehabilitation and prohibit the return to full activity.

ELBOW EXAMINATION SPECIAL TESTS

In addition to methods discussed in the previous section, including accurate measurement of both distal and proximal joint range of motion, radiographic screening, and muscular strength assessment, several other tests should be included in the comprehensive examination of the athletic elbow. Although it is beyond the scope of this article to completely review all of the necessary tests, several are highlighted based on their overall importance. The reader is referred to Morrey,[50] Ellenbecker and Mattalino,[3] and Magee[51] for more complete articles solely on examination of the elbow.

Clinical testing of the joints proximal and distal to the elbow allows the examiner to rule out referral symptoms and ensure that elbow pain is from a local musculoskeletal origin. Overpressure of the cervical spine in the motions of flexion/extension and lateral flexion/rotation, as well as quadrant or Spurling test[52] combining extension with ipsilateral lateral flexion and rotation, are commonly used to clear the cervical spine and rule out radicular symptoms.[53] Tong and colleagues[52] tested the Spurling maneuver to determine the diagnostic accuracy of this examination maneuver. The Spurling test had a sensitivity of 30% and specificity of 93%. Caution must therefore be used when basing the clinical diagnosis solely on this examination maneuver. The test is not sensitive but is specific for cervical radiculopathy, and can be used to help confirm a cervical radiculopathy.

In addition to clearing the cervical spine centrally, clearing the glenohumeral joint is important. Determining the presence of concomitant impingement or instability is also highly recommended.[3] Use of the Sulcus sign[54] to determine the presence of multidirectional instability of the glenohumeral joint, along with the subluxation/relocation sign[55] and load and shift test, can provide valuable insight into the status of the glenohumeral joint. The impingement signs of Neer[56] and Hawkins and Kennedy[57] are also helpful in ruling out proximal tendon pathology.

In addition to the clearing tests for the glenohumeral joint, full inspection of the scapulothoracic joint is recommended. Clinical experience via observation noted by the authors of this article includes the high association of scapular and rotator cuff weakness with overuse elbow injury in athletes. The presence of overuse injuries in the elbow occurring with proximal injury to the shoulder complex or with scapulothoracic dysfunction is widely reported,[6,17,50] and thus a thorough inspection of the proximal joint is extremely important in the comprehensive management of elbow pathology.

Therefore, removal of the patient's shirt or examination of the patient in a gown with full exposure of the upper back is highly recommended. Kibler and colleagues[58] have recently presented a classification system for scapular pathology. Careful observation of the patient at rest and with the hands placed on the hips, as well as during active overhead movements, is recommended to identify prominence of particular borders of the scapula, as well as a lack of close association with the thoracic wall during movement.[59,60] Bilateral comparison forms the primary basis for identifying scapular pathology; however, in many athletes bilateral scapular pathology can be observed.

Several tests specific for the elbow should be performed to assist in the diagnosis of elbow dysfunction. These tests include the Tinel test, varus and valgus stress tests, milking test, valgus extension overpressure test, bounce home test, provocation tests, and the moving valgus test. The Tinel test involves tapping of the ulnar nerve in the medial region of the elbow, over the cubital tunnel retinaculum. Reproduction of paresthesias or tingling along the distal course of the ulnar nerve indicates irritability of the ulnar nerve.[50]

The valgus stress test is used to evaluate the integrity of the ulnar collateral ligament. The position used for testing the anterior band of the ulnar collateral ligament is characterized by 15° to 25° of elbow flexion and forearm supination. The slight elbow flexion position is used to unlock the olecranon from the olecranon fossa, and decreases the stability provided by the osseous congruity of the joint. This position places a greater relative stress on the medial ulnar collateral ligament.[61] Reproduction of medial elbow pain, in addition to unilateral increases in ulnohumeral joint laxity, indicates a positive test. Grading the test is typically performed using the American Academy of Orthopedic Surgeons guidelines of Grade I 0 to 5 mm, Grade II 5 to 10 mm, and Grade III greater than 10 mm.[34] Use of greater than 25° of elbow flexion will increase the amount of humeral rotation during performance of the valgus stress test will transmit misleading information to the clinician's hands. Safran and colleagues[62] studied the effect of forearm rotation during performance of the valgus stress test of the elbow. These investigators found that laxity of the ulnohumeral joint was always greatest when the elbow was tested with the forearm in neutral rotation compared with either the fully pronated or supinated position.

The milking sign is a test the patient performs on himself, with the elbow in approximately 90° of elbow flexion (**Fig. 3**). By reaching under the involved elbow with the contralateral extremity, the patient grasps the thumb of their injured extremity and pulls in a lateral direction, thus imposing a valgus stress to the flexed elbow. Some patients may not have enough flexibility to perform this maneuver, and a valgus stress can be imparted by the examiner to mimic this movement, which stresses the posterior band of the ulnar collateral ligament.[61]

The varus stress test is performed using similar degrees of elbow flexion and shoulder and forearm positioning. This test assesses the integrity of the lateral ulnar collateral ligament, and should be performed along with the valgus stress test to completely evaluate the medial/lateral stability of the ulnohumeral joint.

The valgus extension overpressure test has been reported by Andrews and colleagues[63] to determine whether posterior elbow pain is caused by a posteromedial osteophyte abutting the medial margin of the trochlea and the olecranon fossa (**Fig. 4**). This test is performed by passively extending the elbow while maintaining a valgus stress to the elbow. This test is meant to simulate the stresses imparted to the posterior medial part of the elbow during the acceleration phase of the throwing or serving motion. Reproduction of pain in the posteromedial aspect of the elbow indicates a positive test.

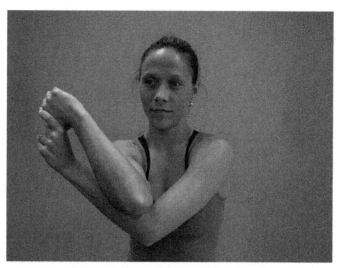

Fig. 3. Milking sign for evaluation of the ulnar collateral ligament.

The use of provocation tests can be applied when screening the muscle tendon units of the elbow. Provocation tests consist of manual muscle tests to determine pain reproduction. The specific tests used to screen the elbow joint of a patient with suspected elbow pathology include wrist and finger flexion and extension, as well as forearm pronation and supination.[64] These tests can be used to provoke the muscle tendon unit at the lateral or medial epicondyle. Testing of the elbow at or near full extension can often recreate localized lateral or medial elbow pain secondary to tendon degeneration.[19] Reproduction of lateral or medial elbow pain with resistive muscle testing (provocation testing) may indicate concomitant tendon injury at the elbow, and would direct the clinician to perform a more complete elbow examination.

One of the more recent elbow special tests reported in the literature is the moving valgus test.[65] This test is performed with the patient's upper extremity in approximately 90° of abduction (**Fig. 5**). The elbow is maximally flexed, and a moderate valgus stress is imparted to the elbow to simulate the late cocking phase of the throwing motion.[1] Maintaining the modest valgus stress at the elbow, the elbow is extended from the fully flexed position. A positive test for ulnar collateral ligament injury is confirmed when reproduction of the patient's pain occurs and is maximal over the medial ulnar collateral ligament between 120° and 70° in what the investigators have termed the "shear angle" or pain zone. O'Driscoll and colleagues[65] examined 21 athlete patients with a primary complaint of medial elbow pain from medial collateral ligament insufficiency or other valgus overload abnormality using the moving valgus test. The moving valgus test was found to be highly sensitive (100%) and specific (75%) when compared with arthroscopic exploration of the medial ulnar collateral ligament. The mean angle of maximum pain reproduction in this study was 90° of elbow flexion. This test can provide valuable clinical input during the evaluation of the patient with medial elbow pain.

These special examination techniques are unique to the elbow and, when combined with a thorough examination of the upper extremity kinetic chain and cervical spine, can result in an objectively based assessment of the patient's pathology and enable the clinician to design a treatment plan based on the examination findings.

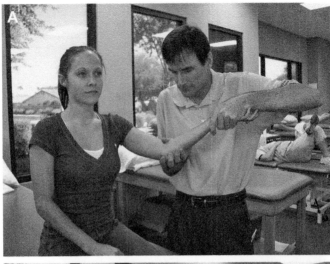

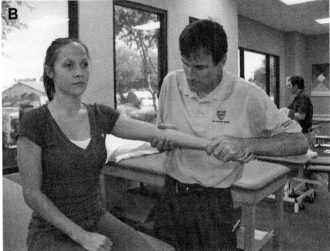

Fig. 4. (*A, B*), Valgus extension overpressure test.

TREATMENT

The treatment of overuse elbow injuries such as humeral epicondlylitis begins following the thorough evaluation and referral to physical therapy. Patients initially are treated to reduce pain, and increase range of motion, muscular strength, and overall function of the injured upper extremity. As mentioned earlier, the entire upper extremity kinetic chain is evaluated and is also integrated into the treatment process. For the purposes of this article, several key concepts are covered encompassing the treatment of the injured athlete's elbow. These concepts include understanding the treatment basis for tendonitis versus tendonosis, a very important distinction for the treatment of humeral epicondlylitis, as discussed earlier in this article.[19] In addition, the important concepts of rotator cuff and scapular stabilization, often viewed as only applicable for the treatment of shoulder dysfunction, are outlined as they

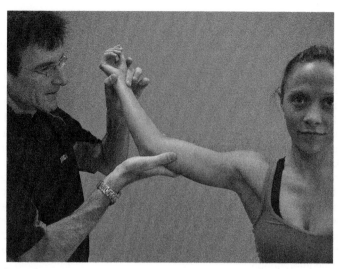

Fig. 5. Moving valgus test.

form an extremely important base for the treatment of the distal upper extremity. Finally, exercise progressions for the distal upper extremity and return to activity guidelines are discussed.

Treatment of Tendonitis Versus Tendonosis

Lateral epicondylitis represents a frequent overuse injury.[66,67] Wilson and Best[68] state that there is a common misconception that symptomatic tendon injuries are inflammatory: because of this, these injuries often are mislabeled as "tendonitis." Acute inflammatory tendinopathies exist, but many patients will have chronic symptoms suggesting a degenerative condition that should be labeled as "tendinosus" or "tendinopathy." Stasinopoulos and Johnson[69] reported a plethora of terms that have been used to describe lateral epicondylitis including tennis elbow, epicondylalgia, tendonitis, tendonosis, and tendinopathy. These terms usually have the prefix extensor or lateral elbow. Lateral elbow tendinopathy seems to be the most appropriate term to use in clinical practice because other terms make reference to inappropriate etiologic, anatomic, and pathophysiologic terms. The correct diagnostic term is important for the right treatment.

Zeisig and colleagues[70] and Riley[71] also indicate that tennis elbow with tendonosis of extensor carpi radialis brevis is a condition with unknown etiology and pathogenesis, and difficult to treat. Croisier and colleagues[72] found that despite the many conservative treatment procedures, prolonged symptoms and relapse are frequently observed. Most treatment options have yet to undergo evaluation for efficacy in well-designed clinical trials, yet there is a generally favorable response to nonoperative or conservative management.[73] Wilson and Best[68] and Gabel[74] indicate that most patients with overuse tendinopathies (about 80%) fully recover within 3 to 6 months. However, 36 years ago Coonrad and Hooper[75] provided an overview of the treatment of tennis elbow. What have clinicians learned in the last 3 and a half decades?

Definitions: Tendonitis and Tendonosis

As stated earlier in this article, several studies[19,76–78] described the histopathological findings showing tennis elbow as a chronic degenerative condition, regeneration, and microtears of the tendonous tissue called tendonosis. Neurochemicals including glutamate, substance P, and calcitonin gene-related peptides have been identified in patients with chronic tennis elbow and in animal models of tendinopathy. Ashe and colleagues[79] indicate new research showing that tendons exhibit areas of degeneration and a distinct lack of inflammatory cells. Tendonosis is consequently degeneration of the collagen tissue due to aging, microtrauma, or vascular compromise. Riley[80] describes the tendon matrix as being maintained by the resident tenocytes, and there is evidence of a continuous process of matrix remodeling, although the rate of turnover varies at different sites. A change in remodeling activity is associated with the onset of tendinopathy and some changes are consistent with repair, but they may also be an adaptive response to changes in mechanical loading. In addition, repeated minor strain is thought to be the major precipitating factor in tendinopathy. Metalloproteinase enzymes have an important role in the tendon matrix, and the role of these enzymes in tendon pathology is unknown; further work is required to identify novel and specific molecular targets for therapy. Riley also states that the neuropeptides and other factors released by stimulated cells or nerve endings in or around the tendon might influence matrix turnover, and could provide novel targets for therapeutic intervention.

Alfredson and Ohberg,[81] using color Doppler examination, showed structural tendon changes with hypoechoic areas and a local neovascularization, corresponding to the painful area. These investigators demonstrated that treatment with sclerosing injections, targeting the area with neovessels, has the potential to cure the pain in the tendons and also allow patients to go back to full patellar tendon loading activity. Ohberg and Alfredson[82] examined the occurrence of neovascularization before and after eccentric training in the Achilles tendon. After 12 weeks of painful eccentric calf muscle training there was a more normal tendon structure, and in the majority of the tendons there was no remaining neovascularization.

In addition, Ohberg and colleagues[83] performed a 12-week eccentric calf muscle training program. Using ultrasonographic follow-up of patients with mid-portion painful chronic Achilles tendonosis treated with eccentric calf muscle training showed a localized decrease in tendon thickness and a normalized tendon structure in most patients. Remaining structural tendon abnormalities seemed to be associated with residual pain in the tendon. Fredberg and Stengaard-Pedersen[77] state that although the prevailing opinion is that no histologic evidence of acute inflammation has been documented, in newer studies using immunohistochemistry and flow cytometry inflammatory cells have been detected. The "tendonitis myth" consequently needs to continue to be pursued and answered. Therefore, the existing data indicate that the initiators of the tendinopathic pathway include many proinflammatory agents. Because of the complex interaction between the classic proinflammatory agents and neuropeptides, it seems impossible and somewhat irrelevant to distinguish between chemical and neurogenic inflammation. Furthermore, glucocorticoids are, at the moment, an effective treatment in tendinopathy with regard to reduction of pain, tendon thickness, and neovascularization. Fredberg and Stengaard-Pedersen indicate that an inflammatory process may be related not only to the development of tendinopathy but also chronic tendinopathy.

Clinical Presentation: Clusters of Signs and Symptoms in Tendonitis versus Tendonosis

Wilson and Best[68] describe many of the clinical findings as follows. The natural history is gradually increasing load-related localized pain coinciding with increased activity. The examination should check for the signs of inflammation (swelling, pain, erythema, and heat) that would indicate a tendonitis response, asymmetry, range of motion testing, palpation for tenderness, and examination maneuvers that simulate tendon loading and reproduce pain. Despite the absence of inflammation, patients with tennis elbow still present with pain. Zeisig and colleagues[70] have suggested the pain involves a neurogenic inflammation mediated via the neuropeptide Substance P. Furthermore, the area with vascularity found in the extensor origin seems to be related to pain. Most likely, the findings correspond with the vasculoneural ingrowth that has been demonstrated in other painful tendonosis conditions. Struijs and colleagues[84] evaluated the predictive value of diagnostic sonography for the effectiveness of conservative treatment of tennis elbow. However, the use of sonography for the detection of abnormalities in this study demonstrated limited value.

There is no consensus regarding the optimum treatment for tendonitis versus tendonosis. Paoloni and colleagues[85] indicated that no treatment has been universally successful. Nirschl[4] and Nirschl and Ashman[86] indicate that the primary goal of nonsurgical treatment is to revitalize the unhealthy tissue that produces pain. Revascularization and collagen repair of the pathologic tissue is the key to a successful rehabilitation program. These investigators state that successful nonsurgical treatment involves rehabilitative resistance exercises and progression of the exercise program. A variety of treatment interventions have been reported in the literature, including hypospray,[87] topical nitric oxide,[85] oxygen free radicals,[88] ice,[89] phonophoresis and ultrasound,[90] low-level laser,[91–93] extracorporeal shock wave therapy,[94–97] deep transverse friction massage (DTFM),[98] manipulation and mobilization,[99,100] acupuncture, bracing, orthotics,[100,101] combined low-level laser and plyometrics,[91] eccentric training programs,[102,103] eccentric isokinetic program,[72] and a combined exercise program.[68,104,105]

Additional Treatments for Tennis Elbow

Forty years ago, Hughes and Currey[87] described the use of hypospray as a treatment of tennis elbow. An instrument capable of injecting a fine spray of liquid (25 mg hydrocortisone acetate) through intact skin to a depth comparable with an intramuscular injection was the mode of treatment for lateral elbow tendinopathy (LET). Paoloni and colleagues,[85] in a well-designed study, demonstrated that the application of topical nitric oxide improved early pain with activity, late functional measures, and outcomes of patients with LET. Murrell[88] recently described the effectiveness of randomized, controlled clinical trials (RCTs) evaluating the efficacy on nitric oxide donation via a patch in the management of tendinopathy. Manias and Stasinopoulos[89] used ice as a supplement to an exercise program that has been recommended for the management of LET. Ice was used as a supplement along with eccentric exercises and stretching in a rehabilitation program. There were no significant differences in the magnitudes of reduction between the groups at the end of treatment and at the 3-month follow up. However, because of the confounding variables with multiple treatment interventions, it is difficult to determine the efficacy. Klaiman and colleagues[90] demonstrated that ultrasound results in decreased pain and increased pressure tolerance in selected soft tissue injuries. The addition of phonophoresis with fluocinonide does not augment the benefits of ultrasound alone.

Bjordal and colleagues[93] performed a systematic review and meta-analysis for low-level laser therapy (LLLT) in LET. Twelve RCTs satisfied the methodological inclusion criteria. LLLT administered with optimal doses of 904 nm and possibly 632 nm wavelengths directly to the lateral elbow tendon insertions seem to offer short-term pain relief and less disability in LET, both alone and in conjunction with an exercise regimen. Stasinopoulos and Johnson[106] used a qualitative analysis of 9 studies that met the inclusion criteria. Poor results were revealed as to the effectiveness of LLLT for LET because it is a dose-response modality, and the optimal treatment dosage has not been identified.

Rompe and colleagues[94] performed an RCT and found that eccentric loading showed inferior results to low-energy shock wave therapy as applied in patients with chronic recalcitrant tendinopathy of the insertion of the Achilles tendon. Wang and colleagues[107] demonstrated that extracorporeal shock wave therapy appeared to be more effective and safer than traditional conservative treatments in the management of patients with chronic patellar tendinopathy.

Rompe and Maffulli[95] performed a qualitative study-by-study assessment that was thought to be of greater relevance than a pooled meta-analysis of statistically and clinically heterogeneous data of RCTs, which are difficult to interpret. This study included 10 trials that included 948 participants. In a qualitative systematic per-study analysis identifying common and diverging details of 10 RCTs, evidence was found for effectiveness of shock wave treatment for tennis elbow under well-defined, restrictive conditions only.

Brosseau and colleagues,[98] in their Cochrane review, determined that DTFM combined with other physiotherapy modalities did not show consistent benefit over the control of pain, improvement of grip strength, and functional status for patients with extensor carpi radialis tendonitis (ECRT). Low-level laser and plyometrics were more effective using a variety of outcome measures than plyometrics by themselves for treatment of lateral epicondylitis.[91] Stergioulas and colleagues,[92] in a Level I RCT study, found that LLLT accelerated clinical recovery from chronic Achilles tendinopathy when added to an eccentric exercise regimen.

Eccentric Training Programs

One specific variable studied with specific regard to treatment of tendon pathology is the use of eccentric exercise. There is limited research regarding the efficacy of eccentric overload training with LET and treatment of other tendon overuse injuries. Kingma and colleagues[108] performed a systematic review of eccentric overload training in patients with chronic Achilles tendinopathy. Nine clinical trials met the inclusion criteria. The included trials showed an improvement in pain after eccentric overload training. However, because of the methodological shortcomings of the trials, no definite conclusion can be drawn concerning the effects of eccentric overload training. Although the effects of eccentric exercise training in tendinopathy on pain are promising, the magnitude of the effects cannot be determined. Knobloch,[103] using a laser Doppler system for capillary blood flow, tissue oxygen saturation, and postcapillary venous filling pressure, evaluated the tendon's microcirculation in response to a 12-week daily painful home-based eccentric training regimen (3 × 15 repetitions per tendon each day). Knobloch found that daily eccentric training for Achilles tendinopathy is a safe and easy measure, with beneficial effects on the microcirculatory tendon levels without any adverse effects in both mid-portion and insertional Achilles tendinopathy. Malliaras and colleagues[102] performed a MEDLINE database search on eccentric training programs for LET. Their results demonstrated that eccentric training in the management of LET has demonstrated encouraging results, although the literature is limited and eccentric programs are varied.

Combined Exercise Programs

Stasinopoulos and colleagues[105] described the use and effects of strengthening and stretching exercise programs in the treatment of LET. These investigators recommend slow progressive eccentric exercises being performed with the elbow in extension, forearm in pronation, and wrist in an extended position. However, they admit the details regarding speed of loading and the details (reps, sets, volume) of the eccentric exercise programs have not been defined. Stasinopoulos and colleagues also recommended static stretching exercises to the lateral muscle tendon unit (MTU) before and after the eccentric exercises for 30 to 45 seconds with a 30-second rest interval between each procedure. However, the details of the optimum parameters for treating LET have yet to be elucidated in a well-designed trial.

There are a few systematic reviews using eccentric exercises in treating patients with lower extremity tendonosis.[109,110] Wasielewski and Kotsko[109] reviewed 11 studies in their systematic review, and the methodological score was 5.3 out of 10 based on the PEDro criteria. Based on the best evidence available, it seems that eccentric exercise may reduce pain and improve strength in lower extremity tendonosis, but whether eccentric exercise is more effective than other forms of therapeutic exercise for the resolution of tendonosis symptoms remains questionable. Woodley and colleagues[110] evaluated 20 relevant studies using the PEDro scale, which included treating lower and upper extremity tendinopathies. These investigators reached a similar conclusion, which demonstrates the dearth of high-quality research in support of the clinical effectiveness of eccentric exercise over other treatments in the management of tendinopathies.

Rotator Cuff and Scapular Stabilization

In addition to the use of therapeutic modalities and eccentric exercise to directly address the injured tendon at the elbow, the use of proximal stabilization and exercise techniques are also warranted during the treatment of the athlete with overuse elbow injury. Several key scapular strengthening exercises that target strengthening of the lower trapezius and serratus anterior force couple are recommended.[111] Scapular stabilization exercises are emphasized, and include external rotation with retraction (**Fig. 6**), an exercise shown to recruit the lower trapezius at a rate 3.3 times more than the upper trapezius and use the important position of scapular retraction.[112] Multiple seated rowing variations are recommended. These variants include the

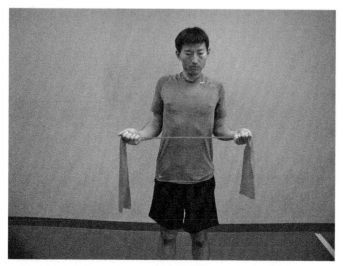

Fig. 6. External rotation with scapular retraction with elastic resistance.

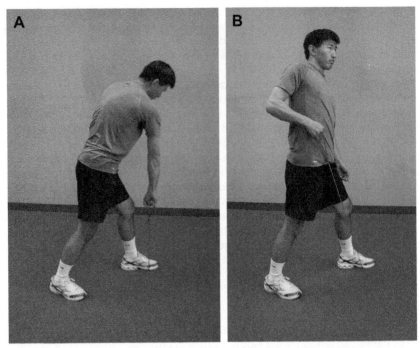

Fig. 7. (*A, B*), Lawn mower exercise for scapular stabilization using elastic resistance.

lawn mower exercise (**Fig. 7**) and low row variations, which have been studied with EMG quantification by Kibler and colleagues.[113]

Progression to closed chain exercise using the "plus" position, which is characterized by maximal scapular protraction, has been recommended by Moesley and colleagues[114] and Decker and colleagues[115] for its inherent maximal serratus anterior

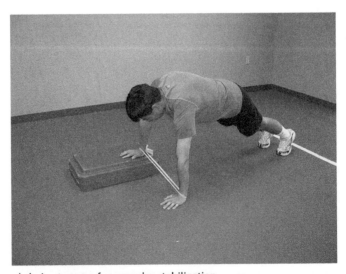

Fig. 8. Closed chain step-ups for scapular stabilization.

1. SIDELYING EXTERNAL ROTATION:
Lie on uninvolved side, with involved arm
at side, with a small pillow between arm
and body. Keeping elbow of involved arm bent
and fixed to side, raise arm into external
rotation. Slowly lower to starting position
and repeat.

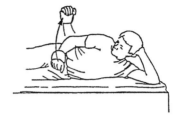

2. SHOULDER EXTENSION:
Lie on table on stomach, with involved arm
hanging straight to the floor. With thumb
pointed outward, raise arm straight back into
extension toward your hip. Slowly lower
arm and repeat.

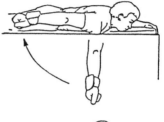

3. PRONE HORIZONTAL ABDUCTION:
Lie on table on stomach, with involved arm
hanging straight to the floor. With thumb
pointed outward, raise arm out to the side,
parallel to the floor. Slowly lower arm,
and repeat.

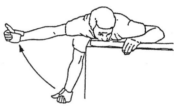

4. 90/90 EXTERNAL ROTATION:
Lie on table on stomach, with shoulder
abducted to 90 degrees and arm supported
on table, with elbow bent at 90 degrees.
Keeping the shoulder and elbow fixed,
rotate arm into external rotation, slowly
lower to start position, and repeat.

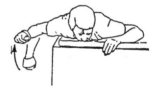

Fig. 9. Rotator cuff exercise movement patterns based on EMG research emphasizing posterior rotator cuff activation and positions with less than 90° of glenohumeral joint elevation.

recruitment. Closed-chain step-ups (**Fig. 8**), and quadruped position rhythmic stabilization and variations of the pointer position (unilateral arm and ipsilateral leg extension weight bearing) are all used in endurance-oriented formats (timed sets of 30 seconds or more) to enhance scapular stabilization. Uhl and colleagues[116] have demonstrated the effects of increasing weight bearing and successive decreases in the number of weight-bearing limbs on muscle activation of the rotator cuff and scapular musculature, and provide guidance for closed-chain exercise progression in the upper extremity.

Strengthening the posterior rotator cuff to provide strength, fatigue resistance, and optimal muscle balance are of paramount importance when working with individuals in this population. **Fig. 9** shows the recommended exercises used by the authors of this article for rotator cuff strengthening. These exercises are based on EMG research showing high levels of posterior rotator cuff activation.[117–120] Use of the prone horizontal abduction exercise is emphasized, as research has shown this position to create high levels of supraspinatus muscular activation,[117,118] making it an alternative to the widely used empty-can exercise that often can cause impingement due to the combined inherent movements of internal rotation and elevation. Three sets of 15 to 20 repetitions are recommended to create a fatigue response and improve local muscular endurance.[121] For application to the patient with elbow dysfunction, these exercises can be performed using a cuff weight attached proximal to the elbow if distal weight attachment provokes pain or stress to the healing elbow structures. Moncreif and colleagues[122] have demonstrated the efficacy of these exercises in a 4-week training paradigm, and measured 8% to 10% increases in isokinetically measured internal and external rotation strength in healthy subjects. These isotonic exercises are coupled with an external rotation exercise with elastic resistance, to provide resistance to the posterior rotator cuff in both a neutral and 90° abducted position in the scapular plane.

Recent research has provided guidance regarding the use of resistive exercise in shoulder rehabilitation. Bitter and colleagues[123] measured EMG activity of the infraspinatus and middle and posterior deltoid during external rotation exercise in healthy subjects. Monitoring of muscular activity occurred during external rotation exercise at 10%, 40%, and 70% activation levels (percentage of maximal). Their important study found increased relative infraspinatus activity when the resistive exercise level was at 40% of maximal effort, indicating more focused activity from the infraspinatus and less compensatory activation of the deltoid. This study confirms that the use of lower intensity strengthening exercises optimizes the activation from the rotator cuff and deemphasizes the input from the deltoid and other prime movers that often occurs with higher intensity resistive loading.

Carter and colleagues[124] studied the effects of an 8-week training program of plyometric upper extremity exercise and external rotation strengthening with elastic resistance. These investigators found increased eccentric external rotation strength, concentric internal rotation strength, and improved throwing velocity in collegiate baseball players, showing the positive effects of plyometric and elastic resistance training in overhead athletes. **Fig. 10** shows a prone 90/90 plyometric that can be used with the athlete maintaining a retracted scapular position with the shoulder in 90° of abduction and 90° of external rotation. The plyo ball is rapidly dropped and

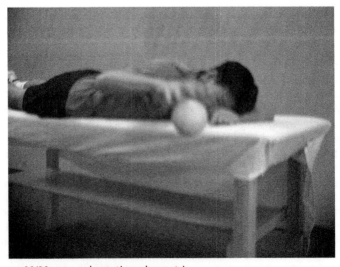

Fig. 10. Prone 90/90 external rotation plyometric.

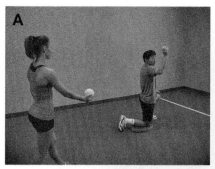
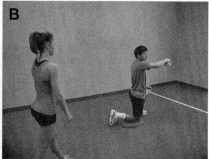
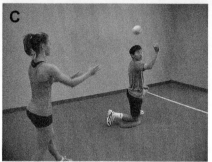

Fig. 11. (*A–C*) Reverse catch plyometric.

caught over a 2- to 3-inch (3 to 6 cm) movement distance for sets of 30 to as much as 40 seconds to address local muscular endurance. **Fig. 11** shows a reverse catch plyometric exercise that is performed again with the glenohumeral joint in the 90/90 position. The ball is tossed from behind the patient to load eccentrically the posterior rotator cuff (external rotators) with a rapid concentric external rotation movement performed as the patient throws the ball back, keeping the abducted position of the shoulder with 90° of elbow flexion. These one-arm plyometric exercises can be preceded by two-arm catches over the shoulder to determine readiness for the one-arm loading. Small 1-pound (0.5 kg) medicine balls or soft weights (Theraband; Hygenic Corporation, Akron, OH) are used initially with progression to 1 to 1.5 kg as the patient progresses in both skill and strength development.

Distal Upper Extremity Exercises for the Adolescent Overhead Athlete

Exercises to improve strength and promote muscular endurance of the forearm and wrist include both traditional curls for the flexors and extensors with either light isotonic dumbbells or elastic tubing or bands, as well as forearm pronation/supination and radioulnar deviation with a counterbalanced weight. Although truly simplistic, these exercises help to provide additional muscular support to the distal extremity, and provide protection and countering to the large forces in this region encountered with both throwing and overhead serving motions.

Due to the anatomic orientation of the flexor carpi ulnaris and flexor digitorum superficialis overlaying the ulnar collateral ligament, isotonic and stabilization activities for these muscles may assist in stabilizing the medial elbow in the overhead throwing athlete.[125] These isotonic exercises with light weights or elastic tubing or bands form the cornerstone of the base program for distal strengthening.[126]

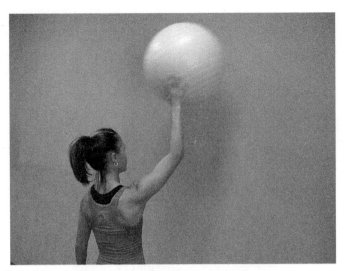

Fig. 12. Ball dribbling for distal upper extremity strengthening.

Integration of more advanced, ballistic type exercises can be recommended for these athletes. Rapid ball dribbling in sets of 30 seconds with a basketball or small physio ball both off the ground and in an elevated position off the wall (**Fig. 12**) are recommended. In addition, specific plyometric drills for the forearm musculature include wrist flexion flips (**Fig. 13**) and wrist flexion snaps (**Fig. 14**). A plyometric exercise used

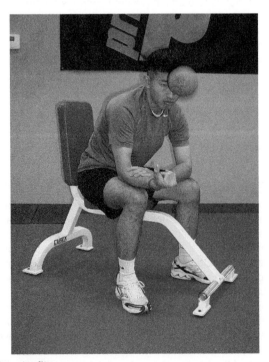

Fig. 13. Plyometric wrist flips.

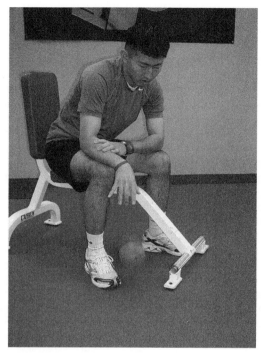

Fig. 14. Plyometric wrist snaps.

in end-stage rehabilitation to provide a valgus overload stress is the internal rotation plyometric in 0° abduction (**Fig. 15**) This exercise can prepare the athlete for throwing activity using a controlled overload stress in the clinical environment. All the plyometric drills constitute an important component of an end-stage rehabilitation program as well as a sport-specific conditioning program for throwing athletes.

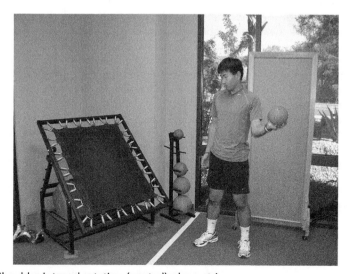

Fig. 15. Shoulder internal rotation (neutral) plyometric.

Return to Sport/Interval Return Programs

Of the phases employed in the rehabilitation process for elbow injury, the return to activity phase is the one that is most frequently ignored or cut short, resulting in serious consequences for reinjury. Objective criteria for entry into this stage are: tolerance of the previously stated resistive exercise series, objectively documented strength equal to the contralateral extremity with either manual assessment (manual muscle testing) or preferably isokinetic testing and isometric strength, distal grip strength measured with a dynamometer, and a functional range of motion. Of note, often in the elite athlete with chronic musculoskeletal adaptations full elbow range of motion is not always attainable, secondary to the osseous and capsular adaptations discussed earlier in this article.

Characteristics of interval sport return programs include alternate day performance, as well as gradual progressions of intensity and repetitions of sport activities. For the interval tennis program, for example, low-compression tennis balls such as the Pro-Penn Star Ball (Penn Racquet Sports, Phoenix, AZ) or foam balls used during the teaching process of tennis to children can be used. These balls are highly recommended for use during the initial phase of the return to tennis program, and result in a decrease in impact stress and increased patient tolerance to the activity. In addition, performing the interval program under supervision, either during therapy or with a knowledgeable teaching professional or coach, allows for the biomechanical evaluation of technique and guards against overzealous intensity levels, which can be a common mistake in well-intentioned, motivated patients. Using the return program on alternate days, with rest between sessions, allows for recovery and decreases the risk of reinjury.

An interval tennis program has been published,[64,127] and the reader is referred to these publications for additional discussion of this important process. In addition, similar concepts are employed in the interval throwing program that has been published previously.[128] Similar to the interval tennis program, having the patient's throwing mechanics evaluated using video and by a qualified coach or biomechanist are very important parts of the return to activity phase of the rehabilitation process.

Two other important aspects of the return to sport activity are the continued application of resistive exercise and the modification or evaluation of the patient's equipment. Continuation of the total arm strength rehabilitation exercises using elastic resistance, medicine balls, and isotonic or isokinetic resistance is important to continue to enhance not only strength but also muscular endurance. Inspection and modification of the patient's tennis racquet or golf clubs is also important. For example, lowering the string tension several pounds and ensuring that the player uses a more resilient or softer string such as a coreless multifilament synthetic string or gut, is widely recommended for tennis players with upper extremity injury histories.[5,6,17] Grip size is also very important, with research showing changes in muscular activity with alteration of handle or grip size.[129] Measurement of proper grip size has been described by Nirschl[6] as corresponding to the distance between the distal tip of the ring finger along the radial border of the finger to the proximal palmar crease. Groppel and Nirschl[130] have also recommended the use of a counterforce brace to decrease stress on the insertion of the flexor and extensor tendons during work or sport activity.

SUMMARY

Treatment of the athlete with an overuse injury requires a thorough evaluation and treatment of the entire upper extremity kinetic chain. Although there are many options available to address elbow pain in the early stages of the rehabilitation process, current evidence is limited as to the identification of a superior modality or series of modalities to attain this important initial goal. The use of an exercise-based approach for the entire upper extremity kinetic chain is recommended, along with a return to a sport program based on objective testing to ensure patient readiness to minimize the effects of reinjury.

REFERENCES

1. Fleisig GS, Andrews JR, Dillman CJ, et al. Kinetics of baseball pitching with implications about injury mechanisms. Am J Sports Med 1995;23:233.
2. Rhu KN, McCormick J, Jobe FW, et al. An electromyographic analysis of shoulder function in tennis players. Am J Sports Med 1988;16:481–5.
3. Ellenbecker TS, Mattalino AJ. The elbow in sport. Champaign (IL): Human Kinetics Publishers; 1997.
4. Nirschl RP, Rodin DM, Ochiai DH, et al. Iontophoretic administration of dexamethasone sodium phosphate for acute epicondylitis: a randomized, double blind, placebo controlled study. Am J Sports Med 2003;31(2):189–95.
5. Nirschl R, Sobel J. Conservative treatment of tennis elbow. Phys Sportsmed 1981;9:43–54.
6. Ollivierre CO, Nirschl RP. Tennis elbow: current concepts of treatment and rehabilitation. Sports Med 1996;22(2):133–9.
7. Carroll R. Tennis elbow: incidence in local league players. Br J Sports Med 1981;15:250–5.
8. Kamien M. A rational management of tennis elbow. Sports Med 1990;9:173–91.
9. Kitai E, Itay S, Ruder A, et al. An epidemiological study of lateral epicondylitis in amateur male players. Ann Chir Main 1986;5:113–21.
10. Hang YS, Peng SM. An epidemiological study of upper extremity injury in tennis players with particular reference to tennis elbow. J Formos Med Assoc 1984;83: 307–16.
11. Priest JD, Jones HH, Tichenor CJC, et al. Arm and elbow changes in expert tennis players. Minn Med 1977;60:399–404.
12. Winge S, Jorgensen U, Nielsen AL. Epidemiology of injuries in Danish championship tennis. Int J Sports Med 1989;10:368–71.
13. Runge F. Zur genese unt behand lung bes schreibekramp fes. Berl Klin Woschenschr 1873;10:245.
14. Cyriax JH, Cyriax PJ. Illustrated manual of orthopaedic medicine. London: Butterworth; 1983.
15. Goldie I. Epicondylitis lateralis humeri. Acta Chir Scand Suppl 1964;339:1.
16. Leadbetter WB. Cell matrix response in tendon injury. Clin Sports Med 1992;11: 533–79.
17. Nirschl RP. Elbow tendinosis/tennis elbow. Clin Sports Med 1992;11:851–70.
18. Nirschl RP, Ashman ES. Tennis elbow tendinosis (epicondylitis). Instr Course Lect 2004;53:587–98.
19. Kraushaar BS, Nirschl RP. Tendinosus of the elbow (tennis elbow). Clinical features and findings of histopathological, immunohistochemical and electron microscopy studies. J Bone Joint Surg Am 1999;81:259–78.
20. Wilson FD, Andrews JR, Blackburn TA. Valgus extension overload in the pitching elbow. Am J Sports Med 1983;11(2):83–8.
21. Bennett GE. Elbow and shoulder lesions of baseball players. Am J Surg 1959; 98:484–92.

22. Indelicato PA, Jobe FW, Kerlan RK, et al. Correctable elbow lesions in professional baseball players: a review of 25 cases. Am J Sports Med 1979;7:72–5.

23. Slocum DB. Classification of the elbow injuries from baseball pitching. Am J Sports Med 1978;6:62.

24. Joyce ME, Jelsma RD, Andrews JR. Throwing injuries to the elbow. Sports Med Arthrosc 1995;3:224–36.

25. Wolf BR, Altchek DW. Elbow problems in elite tennis players. Tech Shoulder Elbow Surg 2003;4(2):55–68.

26. Morrey BF. The elbow and its disorders. Philadelphia: Elsevier; 1998.

27. Kobayashi K, Burton KJ, Rodner C, et al. Lateral compression injuries in the pediatric elbow: Panner's disease and osteochondritis dissecans of the capitellum. J Am Acad Orthop Surg 2004;12(4):246–54.

28. Auvinen JP, Tammelin TH, Taimela SP, et al. Musculoskeletal pains in relation to different sport and exercise activities in youth. Med Sci Sports Exerc 2008; 40(11):1890–900.

29. Graviss ER, Hoffman AD. Imaging of the pediatric elbow. In: Morrey BF, editor. The elbow and its disorders. 2nd edition. Philadelphia: WB Saunders; 1993. p. 181–8.

30. Salter RB, Harris WR. Injuries involving the epiphyseal plate. J Bone Joint Surg Am 1963;45:587–632.

31. Kibler WB. Clinical biomechanics of the elbow in tennis. Implications for evaluation and diagnosis. Med Sci Sports Exerc 1994;26:1203–6.

32. King JW, Brelsford HJ, Tullos HS. Analysis of the pitching arm of the professional baseball pitcher. Clin Orthop Relat Res 1969;67:116–23.

33. Chinn CJ, Priest JD, Kent BE. Upper extremity range of motion, grip strength, and girth in highly skilled tennis players. Phys Ther 1974;54:474–82.

34. Ellenbecker TS, Mattalino AJ, Elam EA, et al. Medial elbow laxity in professional baseball pitchers: a bilateral comparison using stress radiography. Am J Sports Med 1998;26(3):420–4.

35. Wright RW, Steeger May K, Wasserlauf BI, et al. Elbow range of motion in professional baseball pitchers. Am J Sports Med 2006;34(2):190–3.

36. Glousman RE, Barron J, Jobe FW, et al. An electromyographic analysis of the elbow in normal and injured pitchers with medial collateral ligament insufficiency. Am J Sports Med 1992;20:311–7.

37. Dines JS, Frank JB, Akerman M, et al. Glenohumeral internal rotation deficits in baseball players with ulnar collateral ligament deficiency. Am J Sports Med 2009;37(3):566–70.

38. Ellenbecker TS, Roetert EP, Bailie DS, et al. Glenohumeral joint total rotation range of motion in elite tennis players and baseball pitchers. Med Sci Sports Exerc 2002;34(12):2052–6.

39. Borsa PA, Dover GC, Wilk KE, et al. Glenohumeral range of motion and stiffness in professional baseball pitchers. Med Sci Sports Exerc 2006;38(1):21–6.

40. Roetert EP, Ellenbecker TS, Brown SW. Shoulder internal and external rotation range of motion in nationally ranked junior tennis players: a longitudinal analysis. J Strength Cond Res 2000;14(2):140–3.

41. Kibler WB, Chandler TJ, Livingston BP, et al. Shoulder range of motion in elite tennis players. Am J Sports Med 1996;24(3):279–85.

42. Priest JD, Jones HH, Nagel DA. Elbow injuries in highly skilled tennis players. J Sports Med 1974;2(3):137–49.

43. Waslewski GL, Lund P, Chilvers M, et al. MRI evaluation of the ulnar collateral ligament of the elbow in asymptomatic, professional baseball players. Paper presented at the AOSSM Meeting. Orlando, Florida, 2002.

44. Rijke AM, Goitz HT, McCue FC. Stress radiography of the medial elbow ligaments. Radiology 1994;191:213–6.
45. Ellenbecker TS. A total arm strength isokinetic profile of highly skilled tennis players. Isokinet Exerc Sci 1991;1:9–21.
46. Kulund DN, Rockwell DA, Brubaker CE. The long term effects of playing tennis. Phys Sportsmed 1979;7:87–92.
47. Ellenbecker TS, Roetert EP. Isokinetic profile of elbow flexion and extension strength in elite junior tennis players. J Orthop Sports Phys Ther 2003;33(2): 79–84.
48. Ellenbecker TS, Roetert EP. Age specific isokinetic glenohumeral internal and external rotation strength in elite junior tennis players. J Sci Med Sport 2003; 6(1):63–70.
49. Wilk KE, Arrigo CA, Andrews JR. Rehabilitation of the elbow in the throwing athlete. J Orthop Sports Phys Ther 1993;17:305–17.
50. Morrey BF. The elbow and its disorders. 2nd edition. Philadelphia: Saunders; 1993.
51. Magee DJ. Orthopedic physical assessment. 3rd edition. Philadelphia: Saunders; 1997.
52. Tong HC, Haig AJ, Yamakawa K. The Spurling test and cervical radiculopathy. Spine 2002;27(2):156–9.
53. Gould JA. The spine. In: Gould JA, Davies GJ, editors. Orthopaedic and sports physical therapy. St Louis (MO): Mosby; 1985.
54. McFarland EG, Torpey BM, Carl LA. Evaluation of shoulder laxity. Sports Med 1996;22:264–72.
55. Jobe FW, Kivitne RS. Shoulder pain in the overhand or throwing athlete. Orthop Rev 1989;18:963–75.
56. Neer CS. Impingement lesions. Clin Orthop 1983;173:70–7.
57. Hawkins RJ, Kennedy JC. Impingement syndrome in athletes. Am J Sports Med 1980;8:151–8.
58. Kibler WB, Uhl TL, Maddux JWQ, et al. Qualitative clinical evaluation of scapular dysfunction: a reliability study. J Shoulder Elbow Surg 2002;11:550–6.
59. Kibler WB. Role of the scapula in the overhead throwing motion. Contemp Orthop 1991;22(5):525–32.
60. Kibler WB. The role of the scapula in athletic shoulder function. Am J Sports Med 1998;26(2):325–37.
61. Morrey B, An KN. Articular and ligamentous contributions to the stability of the elbow joint. Am J Sports Med 1983;11:315–9.
62. Safran MR, McGarry MH, Shin S, et al. Effects of elbow flexion and forearm rotation on valgus laxity of the elbow. J Bone Joint Surg Am 2005;87(9):2065–74.
63. Andrews JR, Wilk KE, Satterwhite YE, et al. Physical examination of the thrower's elbow. J Orthop Sports Phys Ther 1993;6:296–304.
64. Ellenbecker TS. Rehabilitation of shoulder and elbow injuries in tennis players. Clin Sports Med 1995;14(1):87–110.
65. O'Driscoll SW, Lawton RL, Smith AM. The "moving valgus stress test" for medial collateral ligament tears of the elbow. Am J Sports Med 2005;33(2):231–9.
66. Eygendaal D, Rahussen FT, Diercks RL. Biomechanics of the elbow joint in tennis players and relation to pathology. Br J Sports Med 2007;41:820–3.
67. Maffulli N, Wong J, Almekinders LC. Types and epidemiology of tendinopathy. Clin Sports Med 2003;22:675–92.
68. Wilson JJ, Best TM. Common overuse tendon problems: a review and recommendations for treatment. Am Fam Physician 2005;72:811–8.

69. Stasinopoulos D, Johnson MI. "Lateral elbow tendinopathy" is the most appropriate diagnostic term for the condition commonly referred-to as lateral epicondylitis. Med Hypotheses 2006;67:1400–2.
70. Zeisig E, Ohberg L, Alfredson H. Extensor origin vascularity related to pain in patients with tennis elbow. Knee Surg Sports Traumatol Arthrosc 2006;14:659–63.
71. Riley G. Chronic tendon pathology: molecular basis and therapeutic implications. Expert Rev Mol Med 2005;7:1–25.
72. Croisier JL, Foidart-Dessalle M, Tinant F, et al. An isokinetic eccentric programme for the management of chronic lateral epicondylar tendinopathy. Br J Sports Med 2007;41:269–75.
73. Wainstein JL, Nailor TE. Tendinitis and tendinosis of the elbow, wrist and hands. Clin Occup Environ Med 2006;5:299–322.
74. Gabel GT. Acute and chronic tendinopathies at the elbow. Curr Opin Rheumatol 1999;11:138–43.
75. Coonrad RW, Hooper WR. Tennis elbow: its course, natural history, conservative and surgical management. J Bone Joint Surg Am 1973;55:1177–82.
76. Fedorczyk JM. Tennis elbow: blending basic science with clinical practice. J Hand Ther 2006;19:146–53.
77. Fredberg U, Stengaard-Pedersen K. Chronic tendinopathy tissue pathology, pain mechanisms, and etiology with a special focus on inflammation. Scand J Med Sci Sports 2008;18:3–15.
78. Dunn JH, Kim JJ, Davis L, et al. Ten-14 year follow-up on the Nirschl surgical procedure for lateral epicondylitis. Am J Sports Med 2008;36(2):261–6.
79. Ashe MC, McCauley T, Khan KM. Tendinopathies in the upper extremity: a paradigm shift. J Hand Ther 2004;17:329–34.
80. Riley G. Tendinopathy—from basic science to treatment. Nat Clin Pract Rheumatol 2008;4:82–9.
81. Alfredson H, Ohberg L. Neovasculaization in chronic painful patellar tendinosis—promising reulsts after sclerosing neovessels outside the tendon challenge the need for surgery. Knee Surg Sports Traumatol Arthrosc 2005;13:74–80.
82. Ohberg L, Alfredson H. Effects of neovascularization behind the good results with eccentric training in chronic mid-portion Achilles tendinosis? Knee Surg Sports Traumatol Arthrosc 2004;12:465–70.
83. Ohberg L, Lorentzon R, Alfredson H. Eccentric training in patients with chronic Achilles tendinosis: a normalized tendon structure and decreased thickness at follow up. Br J Sports Med 2004;38:8–11.
84. Struijs PA, Spruyt M, Assendelft WJ, et al. The predictive value of diagnostic sonography for the effectiveness of conservative treatment of tennis elbow. AJR Am J Roentgenol 2005;185:1113–8.
85. Paoloni JA, Appleyard RC, Nelson J, et al. Topical nitric oxide application in the treatment of chronic tendinosis at the elbow: a randomized, double-blinded, placebo controlled clinical trial. Am J Sports Med 2003;31:915–20.
86. Nirschl RP, Ashman ES. Elbow tendinopathy: tennis elbow. Clin Sports Med 2003;22:813–36.
87. Hughes GR, Currey HL. Hypospray treatment of tennis elbow. Ann Rheum Dis 1969;28:58–62.
88. Murrell GA. Oxygen free radicals and tendon healing. J Shoulder Elbow Surg 2007;16:S208–14.
89. Manias P, Stasinopoulos D. A controlled clinical pilot trial to study the effectiveness of ice as a supplement to the exercise programme for the management of lateral elbow tendinopathy. Br J Sports Med 2006;40:81–5.

90. Klaiman MD, Shrader JA, Danoff JV. Phonophoresis versus ultrasound in the treatment of common musculoskeletal conditions. Med Sci Sports Exerc 1998; 30:1349–55.
91. Stergioulas A. Effects of low-level laser and plyometric exercises in the treatment of lateral epicondylitis. Photomed Laser Surg 2007;25:205–13.
92. Stergioulas A, Stergioula M, Aarskog R, et al. Effects of low-level laser therapy and eccentric exercises in the treatment of recreational athletes with chronic Achilles tendinopathy. Am J Sports Med 2008;36:881–7.
93. Bjordal JM, Lopes-Martins RA, Joensen J, et al. A systematic review with procedural assessments and meta-analysis of low level laser therapy in lateral elbow tendinopathy (tennis elbow). BMC Musculoskelet Disord 2008;9:75.
94. Rompe JD, Furia J, Maffulli N. Eccentric loading compared with shock wave treatment for chronic insertional Achilles tendinopathy. A randomized controlled trial. J Bone Joint Surg Am 2008;90:52–61.
95. Rompe JD, Maffulli N. Repetitive shock wave therapy for lateral tendinopathy (tennis elbow): a systematic and qualitative analysis. Br Med Bull 2007;83: 355–78.
96. Seil R, Wilmes P, Nuhrenborger C. Extracorporeal shock wave therapy for tendinopathies. Expert Rev Med Devices 2006;3:463–70.
97. Sems A, Dimeff R, Iannotti JP. Extracorporeal shock wave therapy in the treatment of chronic tendinopathies. J Am Acad Orthop Surg 2006;14:195–204.
98. Brosseau L, Casimiro L, Milne S, et al. Deep transverse friction massage for treating tendinitis. Cochrane Database Syst Rev 2002;(4):CD003528.
99. Stoddard A. Manipulation of the elbow joint. Physiotherapy 1971;57:259–60.
100. Pfefer MT, Cooper SR, Uhl NL. Chiropractic management of tendinopathy: a literature synthesis. J Manipulative Physiol Ther 2009;32:41–52.
101. Ilfeld FW, Field SM. Treatment of tennis elbow. Use of a special brace. JAMA 1966;195:67–70.
102. Malliaras P, Maffulli N, Garau G. Eccentric training programmes in the management of lateral elbow tendinopathy. Disabil Rehabil 2008;30:1590–6.
103. Knobloch K. Eccentric training in Achilles tendinopathy: is it harmful to tendon microcirculation? Br J Sports Med 2007;41:e2.
104. Stasinopoulos D, Stasinopoulos I. Comparison of effects of exercise programme, pulsed ultrasound, and transverse friction in the treatment of chronic patellar tendinopathy. Clin Rehabil 2004;18:347–52.
105. Stasinopoulos D, Stasinopoulos I, Johnson MI. An exercise program for the management of lateral elbow tendinopathy. Br J Sports Med 2005;39:944–7.
106. Stasinopoulos DI, Johnson MI. Effectiveness of low-level laser therapy for lateral elbow tendinopathy. Photomed Laser Surg 2005;23:425–30.
107. Wang CJ, Ko JY, Chan YS, et al. Extracorporeal shockwave for chronic patellar tendinopathy. Am J Sports Med 2007;35:972–8.
108. Kingma JJ, deKnikker R, Wittink HM, et al. Eccentric overload training in patients with chronic Achilles tendinopathy: a systematic review. Br J Sports Med 2007; 41:E3.
109. Wasielewski NJ, Kotsko KM. Does eccentric exercise reduce pain and improve strength in physically active adults with symptomatic lower extremity tendinosis? A systematic review. J Athl Train 2007;42:409–21.
110. Woodley BL, Newsham-West RJ, Baxter GD. Chronic tendinopathy: effectiveness of eccentric exercise. Br J Sports Med 2007;41:188–98.
111. Bagg SD, Forrest WJ. A biomechanical analysis of scapular rotation during arm abduction in the scapular plane. Arch Phys Med Rehabil 1988;67:238–45.

112. McCabe RA, Tyler TF, Nicholas SJ, et al. Selective activation of the lower trapezius muscle in patients with shoulder impingement [abstract]. J Orthop Sports Phys Ther 2001;31(1):A-45.

113. Kibler WB, Sciascia AD, Uhl TL, et al. Electromyographic analysis of specific exercises for scapular control in early phases of shoulder rehabilitation. Am J Sports Med 2008;36:1789–98.

114. Moesley JB, Jobe FW, Pink M. EMG analysis of the scapular muscles during a shoulder rehabilitation program. Am J Sports Med 1992;20:128.

115. Decker MJ, Hintermeister RA, Faber KJ, et al. Serratus anterior muscle activity during selected rehabilitation exercises. Am J Sports Med 1999;27: 784–91.

116. Uhl TL, Carver TJ, Mattacola CG, et al. Shoulder musculature activation during upper extremity weightbearing exercise. J Orthop Sports Phys Ther 2003;33(3): 109–17.

117. Blackburn TA, McLeod WD, White B, et al. EMG analysis of posterior rotator cuff exercises. Athl Train 1990;25:40.

118. Reinhold MM, Wilk KE, Fleisig GS, et al. Electromyographic analysis of the rotator cuff and deltoid musculature during common shoulder external rotation exercises. J Orthop Sports Phys Ther 2004;34(7):385–94.

119. Townsend H, Jobe FW, Pink M, et al. Electromyographic analysis of the glenohumeral muscles during a baseball rehabilitation program. Am J Sports Med 1991;19:264.

120. Malanga GA, Jenp YN, Growney ES, et al. EMG analysis of shoulder positioning in testing and strengthening the supraspinatus. Med Sci Sports Exerc 1996; 28(6):661–4.

121. Fleck SJ, Kraemer WJ. Designing resistance training programs. Champaign (IL): Human Kinetics Publishers; 1987.

122. Moncrief SA, Lau JD, Gale JR, et al. Effect of rotator cuff exercise on humeral rotation torque in healthy individuals. J Strength Cond Res 2002;16(2):262–70.

123. Bitter NL, Clisby EF, Jones MA, et al. Relative contributions of infraspinatus and deltoid during external rotation in healthy shoulders. J Shoulder Elbow Surg 2007;16(5):563–8.

124. Carter AB, Kaminski TW, Douex AT Jr, et al. Effects of high volume upper extremity plyometric training on throwing velocity & functional strength ratios of the shoulder rotators in collegiate baseball players. J Strength Cond Res 2007;21(1):208–15.

125. Davidson PA, Pink M, Perry J. Functional anatomy of the flexor pronator muscle in group relation to the medial collateral ligament of the elbow. Am J Sports Med 1995;23:245–50.

126. Roetert EP, Ellenbecker TS. Complete conditioning for tennis. Champaign (IL): Human Kinetics Publishers; 2007.

127. Ellenbecker TS, Wilk KE, Reinold MM, et al. Use of interval return programs for shoulder rehabilitation. In: Ellenbecker TS, editor. Shoulder rehabilitation: non operative treatment. New York: Thieme; 2006.

128. Reinold MM, Wilk KE, Reed J, et al. Internal sport programs: guidelines for baseball, tennis, and golf. J Orthop Sports Phys Ther 2002;32:293–8.

129. Adelsberg S. An EMG analysis of selected muscles with rackets of increasing grip size. Am J Sports Med 1986;14:139–42.

130. Groppel JL, Nirschl RP. A biomechanical and electromyographical analysis of the effects of counter force braces on the tennis player. Am J Sports Med 1986;14:195–200.

Rehabilitation of the Wrist and Hand Following Sports Injury

Carrie A. Jaworski, MD[a,b,*], Michelle Krause, PT, ATC[a],
Jennifer Brown, ATC[a]

KEYWORDS

• Hand injury • Wrist injury • Rehabilitation • Return to play

Hand and wrist injuries are some of the most common injuries among athletes. Literature reviews reveal that a rate of between 3% and 9% of all sports injuries involve the hand or wrist.[1] The true incidence is likely unknown, because many injuries go unrecognized or are under-reported by athletes. Of the reported injuries, most hand and wrist injuries seen are overuse injuries (25%–50%) with the percentage of traumatic injuries varying by sport and position.[2] An additional obstacle of many hand and wrist injuries is that they are often inadequately treated or rehabilitated because athletes disregard what they perceive as inconsequential symptoms, and many health care providers are intimidated by the complexity of the hand and wrist. To maximize the recovery of hand and wrist injuries in athletes, sports medicine providers need to understand the "pearls and pitfalls" associated with common sports injuries affecting the hand and wrist, and aggressively attend to the rehabilitation of such injuries.

ANATOMY AND BIOMECHANICS

The complexity of the hand and wrist is a result of the numerous bones, joints, ligaments, and neurovascular structures that course through the small area. By understanding the contents and workings of the hand and wrist, diagnosis and treatment of injuries become much more effective.

[a] Northwestern University Department of Intercollegiate Sports Medicine, 1501 Central Street, Evanston, IL 60208, USA
[b] Department of Family and Community Medicine, Northwestern University Feinberg School of Medicine, 710 N Lake Shore Drive, 4th Floor, Chicago, IL 60611, USA
* Corresponding author. Northwestern University Department of Intercollegiate Sports Medicine, 1501 Central Street, Evanston, IL 60208.
E-mail address: c-jaworski@northwestern.edu (C.A. Jaworski).

Clin Sports Med 29 (2010) 61–80
doi:10.1016/j.csm.2009.09.007
0278-5919/09/$ – see front matter © 2010 Elsevier Inc. All rights reserved.

WRIST

The wrist joint comprises 8 carpal bones with articulations at the radius or ulna prox-imally, and the metacarpals distally. The carpal bones are situated in 2 rows of 4 bones each, with the scaphoid being the functional link between them because it spans both rows. The proximal row consists of the scaphoid, lunate, triquetrum, and pisiform. The distal row contains the trapezium, trapezoid, capitate, and hamate. The distal carpal row controls the position of the scaphoid and thus the lunate. With ulnar deviation, the distal row is displaced ulnarly and the proximal row moves radially. With radial deviation, the distal part of the scaphoid must shift to avoid the radial styloid. This shift accounts for the differences in the total arc of motion (50°) for radial and ulnar devia-tion, with ulnar deviation averaging 35° and radial deviation averaging 15° of the total arc. Wrist flexion and extension relies on the motion of both carpal rows in unison with the total arc of motion averaging approximately 120° in total.[3] Many studies have demonstrated differences in the motion required at the wrist in various sports.[4,5] Basketball, for instance, requires an average of 50° of extension and 70° of flexion in the dominant wrist, versus only a 32° total arc in the nondominant wrist to shoot a free throw. These subtleties need to be accounted for when splinting and operating on athletes in different sports.

The carpal bones are connected to each other by ligaments. Of these ligaments, the strongest are the palmar ligaments coursing from the proximal carpal row to the radius. Next strongest are the dorsal ligaments, which include the scaphoid-trique-trum and distal radius to lunate and triquetrum. The weakest wrist ligaments are the intrinsic ligaments, scapholunate and lunotriquetral; for this reason most wrist insta-bility comes from disruption of these structures.[3]

Within the wrist, there are no true collateral ligaments to stabilize the radial and ulnar sides. Such structures would inhibit the necessary motions of radial and ulnar devia-tion. Several muscles, however, serve as what Schneider refers to as an "adjustable collateral system." These include the extensor carpi ulnaris (ECU) on the ulnar side, and the abductor pollicis longus (APL) and extensor pollicis brevis (EPB) on the radial side.[3]

Ulnar-sided wrist stability is further enhanced by the triangular fibrocartilage complex (TFCC), which originates from the radius and inserts into the base of the ulnar styloid, the base of the fifth metacarpal, and the ulnar carpus. The TFCC is a cushion for the ulnar carpus and the major stabilizer of the distal radioulnar joint (DRUJ).

The dorsal wrist comprises 6 compartments. The first 5 compartments are formed by a dorsal retinaculum with 6 vertical septa that attach at the distal radius. The sixth compartment is a separate tunnel that is made from an infratendinous retinaculum and houses the ECU. This distinctly separate tunnel allows for unrestricted rotation of the ulna during supination and pronation. These retinacular structures prevent the wrist extensors from "bowstringing" during use.[6]

On the volar side, the flexors of the wrist and fingers, and the median nerve and radial artery, are prevented from bowstringing by the thick transverse carpal ligament.

HAND

The stabilizers of the metacarpal phalangeal (MCP) joints are important to the function of the hand. Stability is reliant on the joint capsule, collateral ligaments, accessory collateral ligaments, volar plate, and musculotendinous units.

The collateral ligaments are located laterally with a dorsal position relative to the axis of rotation. This location results in the ligaments being lax when the MCP joint is in extension, and taut with the MCP joint in flexion. This concept is vitally important when casting or splinting the MCP joint because, if the MCP is immobilized in extension, the collaterals will tighten and it will be difficult to achieve full flexion once mobilization is initiated.

The muscles crossing the MCP joints on the flexor surface include the flexor digitorum superficialis (FDS) and the flexor digitorum profundus (FDP). The FDS flexes the proximal interphalangeal (PIP) joint and the FDP flexes the distal interphalangeal (DIP) joint. The interosseous muscles are lateral to the MCP joints and control abduction/adduction of the MCP joints. The lumbricals originate on the volar aspect of the MCP but insert into the lateral bands dorsal to the PIP and DIP joints. They flex the MCP and extend the interphalangeal (IP) joints.

PHALANGES

IP joint motion is a delicate balance of several systems. The collateral and accessory collateral ligaments stabilize the IP joints on their lateral aspects. Unlike the ligaments of the MCP joints, the collateral ligaments are taut in extension and lax in flexion, meaning that, unless contraindicated, IP joints should be splinted in full extension to help prevent flexion contractures (**Fig. 1**).

Flexion of the IP joints is controlled by the FDS and FDP. The FDS splits proximal to the PIP joint, allowing the FDP to become more superficial as it inserts on the distal phalanx to control DIP flexion.

The FDS inserts on the middle phalanx and controls PIP flexion. There are 5 annular pulleys and 3 cruciate pulleys between the MCP and DIP joints to prevent bowstringing of the tendons.

The extensor surface contains the common extensor tendon. It divides into 3 slips after crossing the MCP joint. The central slip inserts on the dorsal middle phalanx where it controls PIP extension. The 2 lateral slips, referred to as the lateral bands, originate from the lumbricals, after which they travel dorsal and lateral to the PIP joint. They rejoin after the PIP to insert as the terminal extensor on the DIP joint.[3]

Testing the individual function of IP motion and the FDS and FDP muscles is an essential component of any thorough hand injury evaluation (see **Fig. 1**).

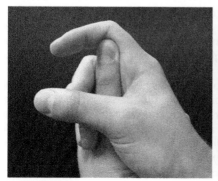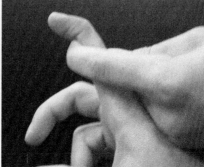

Fig. 1. Blocked PIP and DIP exercises. Stabilizing the proximal phalanx allows the flexion force to concentrate at the PIP joint. When stabilizing the middle phalanx, the flexion force acts at the DIP joint.

WRIST INJURIES
DeQuervain Disease

Anatomy
The tendons and synovial sheaths of the APL and EPB muscles are located in the first dorsal compartment of the wrist. The APL abducts the thumb joint and also functions as a radial deviator of the wrist. The EPB extends the thumb metacarpophalangeal joint and also helps with thumb abduction. The APL and EPB tendons form the radial border of the anatomic snuffbox.

Mechanism of injury
DeQuervain disease, or stenosing tenosynovitis, is the most common wrist tendonitis encountered by athletes.[2] It can be caused by activities that require forceful grasping with ulnar deviation or repetitive thumb use, such as with golf or racquet sports.[7] Repetitive gliding of the APL and EPB tendons beneath the synovial sheath in the first dorsal compartment causes shear microtrauma to the tendons resulting in the signs and symptoms of DeQuervain disease.[2] Less commonly, trauma to the radial styloid or an acute strain can incite the injury.

Recent findings have suggested that DeQuervain disease is often not caused by an inflammatory condition, but a degeneration of the tendon referred to as tendinosis.[8] This may explain why traditional therapeutic approaches to address inflammation are not always successful.

Evaluation findings
The athlete with DeQuervain disease presents with pain over the radial side of the wrist, which can radiate distally or proximally.[9] Pain is typically aggravated by thumb or wrist movements. Resisted thumb extension or abduction can also cause pain, and the patient typically presents with a positive Finklestein test.[8] The Finklestein test is performed by having the patient flex the thumb into the palm while the examiner passively ulnarly deviates the wrist.[2] A test is considered positive if the patient's symptoms of pain are reproduced. The examiner needs to compare with the unaffected side, as this test is uncomfortable.

Management
Nonsurgical management of DeQuervain disease is ideal. Acute treatment of DeQuervain disease includes relative rest, ice, nonsteroidal anti-inflammatory drugs (NSAIDs), and immobilization of the thumb with a thumb spica wrist splint. The traditional type of splint is a radial gutter splint that includes the MCP and carpometacarpal (CMC) joints and wrist. The IP joint of the thumb does not need to be immobilized because the extensor pollicus longus (EPL) is typically not involved. The athlete needs to use the thumb spica splint full time, except for hygiene, for the first 2 to 3 weeks. Wear time can decrease as symptoms abate.

Modalities such as ice, ultrasound, and iontophoresis can be effective in controlling pain and edema. A corticosteroid injection into the first dorsal compartment may provide patients with relief if symptoms persist.[2] It is important to educate the athlete about avoiding aggravating activities, such as heavy grasping or repetitive thumb and wrist motion that increase their pain. The clinician should also look for poor mechanics or weakness proximal to the wrist that may be contributing to the condition.

When conservative treatment fails, surgical release of the first dorsal compartment may be indicated. Complications following surgical release of the first dorsal compartment typically involve injury to superficial and radial nerves, resulting in paresthesia.[2] Scar tissue formation at the incision site may also occur.

Rehabilitation

In nonsurgical cases, the clinician should begin stretching the affected areas through a pain-free range of motion (ROM) once the athlete's pain and swelling has been addressed. Therapy should consist of active and passive ROM exercises, and gentle stretches to promote the gliding of the APL and EPB tendons in the first tunnel. Once pain has decreased, the focus can be on strengthening of the hand, wrist, and thumb musculature. Exercises should begin with isometrics, progress to full ROM against gravity, light weights, and then weight bearing and plyometrics. If symptoms increase at any time, further progression should be delayed.[3]

Rehabilitation following surgical release of the first dorsal compartment can take several months. Patients will typically begin occupational or physical therapy in the weeks following surgery and continue therapy for 6 to 8 weeks, depending on their progress. Initial treatment should address wound care, scar massage, and ROM exercises. As the patient progresses, the strengthening exercises for the hand, thumb, and wrist are introduced, as discussed earlier. Exercises to improve fine motor control and dexterity should also be included, paying special attention to any residual effects from surgery on the superficial and radial nerves.

Return to play

Ideally, the athlete should be pain free with full ROM before returning to activity. Strength should be near normal and be able to protect against further injury. Based on the demands of the particular sport, some athletes can continue to participate with DeQuervain disease before resolution of their pain. Such athletes should be taped or splinted for support while playing and be able to demonstrate no impairment in performance. Low-profile splints can be fashioned to allow for ease of participation. Athletes should also be educated that DeQuervain disease can take a long time to heal, so, by continuing to participate, they need to understand that the time course to complete healing may be further prolonged.

Scaphoid Fracture

Anatomy

The scaphoid is the most commonly fractured carpal bone, accounting for nearly 60% of all carpal injuries, based on its radial-sided location where it spans both carpal rows.[10] The irregularly shaped bone is divided into proximal and distal poles, a tubercle, and a waist.[11] The blood supply to the scaphoid is supplied through the branches of the radial artery, coming distal to proximal.[12] Healing time varies between 6 weeks, for a tuberosity fracture, to up to 20 weeks for a proximal one-third fracture, based on this blood supply distribution. Fractures through the waist of the proximal one-third of the scaphoid are also susceptible to delayed union or avascular necrosis due to its poor blood supply.

Mechanism of injury

The most common mechanism for a scaphoid fracture is falling on an outstretched hand. The scaphoid is susceptible to fracture because it blocks excessive flexion of the wrist.[12] When the wrist hyperextends, the radial styloid often strikes the scaphoid waist, resulting in a fracture.[3] It is also possible to fracture the scaphoid if an axial load is applied to the wrist.[12]

Evaluation findings

Physical examination may reveal limited swelling, but, more commonly, tenderness to palpation in the anatomic snuffbox.[11] The anatomic snuffbox is most visible and palpable when the patient's wrist is in a neutral position and the thumb is extended.

Pain may also be elicited by palpating the scaphoid on the dorsal side of the wrist in extension. Significant swelling may represent a fracture-dislocation. The patient will have almost full wrist ROM, but pain will be elicited with end range flexion and extension.[12]

Management

Initial treatment is centered on confirming the suspected diagnosis of a scaphoid fracture. Initial plain radiographs will frequently not show an acute fracture, making the diagnosis of an acute scaphoid fracture difficult.[4] If a practitioner suspects a scaphoid fracture, the patient should be immobilized in a short-arm thumb spica splint or cast, even if the initial radiograph is negative, to improve healing potential. Repeat films should be taken in 2 weeks, which will then confirm or refute the diagnosis.[11] For competitive athletes, this 2-week waiting period can be frustrating, and a definitive diagnosis may necessitate more advanced imaging, such as a magnetic resonance imaging (MRI) scan, computerized tomography (CT) scan, or bone scan.

Once a diagnosis of scaphoid fracture has been made, the location and type of fracture dictates treatment. Due to the distal-to-proximal blood supply in the scaphoid, a patient with a proximal pole fracture should be referred for possible internal fixation.[11] In addition, if nonunion develops after a normal course of casting, conservative treatment referral is necessary. Regardless of location, a hand surgeon will typically treat all displaced fractures and fracture-dislocations with internal fixation.[4] Nondisplaced fractures are often treated with simple immobilization.[12] The recommended immobilization is obtained through a long-arm cast for 6 weeks and then a short-arm cast, if needed, until healing is achieved. Nondisplaced fractures of the distal third of the scaphoid are expected to result in union after 6 to 8 weeks of immobilization, fractures of the middle third may require 8 to 12 weeks, and proximal third fractures often require 12 to 24 weeks of immobilization.[11] Competitive athletes may wish to discuss potential operative fixation of the fracture with a hand surgeon early on in the process. Surgical intervention has not been proven to speed up the healing process of the fracture, but it may allow for the earlier return to play (RTP) that many athletes desire.[13]

Rehabilitation

Regardless of surgical or nonsurgical treatment of a scaphoid fracture, an exercise program is necessary once the cast is removed. The lengthy immobilization period often results in atrophy of the forearm and decreased ROM of the wrist and thumb.[12] After the cast is discontinued, a removable splint is necessary for exercising. Initially only active range of motion (AROM) is allowed, focusing on wrist flexion, extension, radial and ulnar deviation, and thumb flexion, extension, and opposition. After 1 to 2 weeks, passive range of motion (PROM) is allowed for the same motions.[4] As a therapist begins PROM, putty is used for gentle strengthening. As ROM improves, strengthening activities are increased to include weight training, weight-bearing exercises, plyometrics, and upper-body ergometers for conditioning.[3] The time necessary for a patient to regain full ROM and strength is related to the length of immobilization required. It is necessary to protect the wrist in athletics for at least 3 months after cast removal, and longer if ROM is abnormal and strength is less than 80% of the uninjured side.[12]

RTP

Whether or not an athlete may RTP with a scaphoid fracture is controversial and depends on the sport, athlete, location of the fracture, stability of the fracture, and ability to participate in a cast or splint. If the athlete participates in a noncontact sport and is functional in the cast, RTP is allowed almost immediately. Similarly, athletes treated operatively who participate in noncontact sports can return as soon as initial wound healing has occurred and pain allows.[13] Contact sports present a more difficult situation. Most physicians believe that nonoperative fractures being treated with immobilization should not be allowed to return to contact for 6 weeks so initial healing can occur.[4,13] Once initial healing has occurred, an athlete will need to remain in a playing cast for an additional 6 weeks.[13] Operatively repaired fractures are allowed to return to contact in a playing cast 2 to 3 weeks after surgery.[3] This decreased time away from activity can be attractive to athletes. Once again, surgically and conservatively treated nondisplaced fractures require the same time to heal.[14]

Distal Radius Fracture

Anatomy
Fractures of the distal radius account for one-sixth of all fractures seen in the emergency room, primarily because the radius is slightly longer than the ulna, causing it to extend further distally in the wrist.[15] The distal radius articulates with 3 bones (the scaphoid, lunate, and distal ulna) that result in a spectrum of possible injuries involving the DRUJ, distal ulna, or fracture-dislocations of the carpus. Numerous operative and nonoperative treatments exist, based on the type of fracture, but the overall goal remains the same: a functional wrist and hand.[16]

Mechanism of injury
The most common mechanism for a distal radius fracture is falling on an outstretched hand. The wrist will be extended when contact on the outstretched arm occurs.[12]

Evaluation findings
The athlete will present with pain and swelling in the wrist and there may be obvious ecchymosis and swelling.[12] If apparent deformity is present, capillary refill and a neurovascular screen should be checked.

When diagnosing a distal radius fracture, it is important to be able to determine whether it is extraarticular or intraarticular. Intraarticular fractures can involve the radiocarpal joint, the DRUJ, or both.[11] There is no consensus on how to classify distal radius fractures on a radiograph, with several classification systems in place. Historically, the Frykman classification has been used most often to diagnose the type of fracture[16,17] There are 8 types of fractures; the even numbers indicate an additional fracture of the ulnar styloid. Type I/II are extraarticular; type III/IV are intraarticular, involving the radiocarpal joint; type V/VI are intraarticular involving the radioulnar joint; type VII/VIII are intraarticular involving the radiocarpal and radioulnar joints.[11]

Any type of distal radius fracture that is comminuted or significantly displaced should be referred to an orthopedic surgeon, as these fractures are unstable. In addition, any displaced fracture of types II to VIII should be referred, as it will most likely require surgical intervention and fixation.[12]

Treatment
All distal radius fractures should be reduced and immobilized, even if surgery is indicated.[12] A stable extraarticular fracture can be treated with cast immobilization.[16] Surgically stabilized fractures can involve external fixation, dorsal plating, or volar fixed angle plating, depending on the type of fracture.[6]

Rehabilitation of distal radius fracture
A common complication is wrist and hand stiffness after immobilization, proving how important it is to start ROM early in all uninvolved joints.[3] Regardless of surgical or

nonsurgical intervention, active and passive ROM of the fingers, elbow, shoulder, and rotation of the forearm as early as within 24 hours of intervention is important.[3,16] This motion helps to prevent atrophy of surrounding muscles and tendon adhesions, and creates a muscle pump to aid in the reduction of edema.[3,16] Beginning therapy early after injury also allows for observation to ensure that reduction of the fracture is maintained.[18] If surgical intervention has occurred, wound cleaning may be required of the therapist. By maintaining full shoulder, elbow, and finger ROM, the patient is allowed to focus on the wrist once immobilization ceases, which usually occurs at 6 weeks for nonsurgical cases and 8 weeks after surgical intervention. Active wrist flexion, extension, and radial and ulnar deviation should be done once the cast is removed. (**Figs. 2** and **3**) After about 1 week, PROM begins, including forearm pronation and supination. Once ROM has improved, strengthening begins. A variety of light weights, bands, and tubing are used to increase strength, progressing to weight-bearing exercises such as push-ups, and finally plyometrics.[3,10,18]

RTP

When an athlete with a distal radius fracture is allowed to RTP depends on the type of fracture and their sport. If an athlete has a stable fracture and is casted, they can return once they are pain free, usually at around 2 to 3 weeks. If surgical intervention is necessary, return is usually closer to 6 weeks. With contact-sport athletes, a protective playing cast is necessary for an additional 6 weeks after return. The playing cast can be short-armed, with the wrist in a neutral position, allowing for full thumb, finger, and elbow ROM.[3,10]

TFCC Injuries

Anatomy

As the TFCC is the primary stabilizer of the radioulnar joint, injuries to this ligament can result in significant disability for the athlete. The TFCC is divided into an almost avascular central articular disc component and the dorsal and palmar radioulnar ligaments, which are more vascular and act to stabilize the DRUJ.[4] Traumatic injuries to the TFCC are usually in the periphery, whereas degenerative tears are more often central.

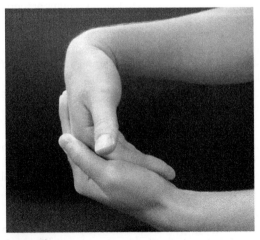

Fig. 2. Wrist extensor stretch.

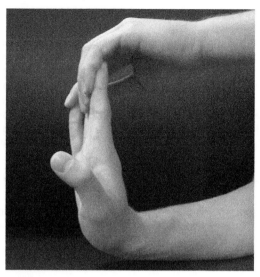

Fig. 3. Wrist flexor stretch.

Mechanism of injury

Acute TFCC injuries can result from a variety of mechanisms. Some examples include a fall on an outstretched hand, a collision on the field of play, landing on or twisting the wrist during a fall, or a bad shot in golf or tennis. Acute injuries may also be superimposed on chronic degenerative changes in sports such as gymnastics, boxing, golf, and in racquet players.[4]

Evaluation findings

Diagnosis of a TFCC injury is often difficult. Any athlete who complains of ulnar-sided wrist pain should be evaluated for a TFCC injury. Pain is usually present with ulnar deviation, extension, and forearm rotation.[3] Tenderness of the TFCC complex is best elicited by palpating the hollow between the ulnar styloid and the pisiform on the ulnar side of the wrist. Several provocative tests can also lead to the diagnosis of a TFCC injury. A positive supination lift test, which is done by having the patient "lift" the examination table with their palms flat on the underside of the table, may suggest a dorsal peripheral tear. One can also have patients attempt to lift themselves off the table, which may provoke ulnar-sided pain or weakness. A positive piano key sign suggests DRUJ instability. This test is done by having the athlete forcibly press both palms into the examination table while the examiner observes for exaggerated dorsal-palmar translation on the injured side. A wrist arthrogram or diagnostic arthroscopy can confirm the diagnosis.

Treatment

Due to the complexity of the TFCC, athletes with these injuries benefit from the expertise of a hand surgeon to determine the most appropriate treatment. Acute injuries with no DRUJ involvement can be treated with immobilization. Injuries to the peripheral regions of the TFCC warrant a more aggressive approach, with surgical repair based on the good vascular supply. Conversely, central tears are more often debrided due to the lack of blood supply. In any situation, early intervention leads to the best result for the athlete.[19]

Rehabilitation of TFCC injuries

In cases that have been debrided, patients are typically splinted for 1 week, and then ROM is started. Strengthening can begin once the athlete has near-normal AROM.[3] Light activity ball contact for golf or tennis athletes may be permitted at 3 weeks, and most return to restricted sports activity at 4 to 6 weeks.[4] Surgical repairs require immobilization that prevents wrist motion and supination and pronation for 4 to 6 weeks. During this time, depending on the surgeon, some will allow supervised active wrist flexion and extension. Once the splint is discontinued, passive ROM can be started. At around 8 to 10 weeks, gentle isometric strengthening can begin, with progression to weight bearing and plyometrics as tolerated. (**Figs. 4** and **5**).

RTP

As with most injuries, RTP is dependent on the sport and position of the athlete. Most can begin aerobic conditioning around the 2-week mark while still wearing a splint. Progression to strength training at around 8 to 10 weeks should include taping for support. Stick-sport athletes may begin stick work around 10 weeks, provided it does not cause pain. Most surgical repairs achieve full RTP at 3 to 4 months.[3,4]

HAND INJURIES
Ulnar Collateral Ligament Sprain (Gamekeeper Thumb)

Anatomy

The MCP joint of the thumb is diarthrodial, which allows for flexion/extension and abduction/adduction. The thumb's MCP ROM is the most variable in the human body and can even vary between the left and the right in the same person.[20] The collateral ligaments provide lateral stability, attach to the lateral condyle of the metacarpal and to the proximal phalanx, and are taut in flexion. The ulnar collateral ligament (UCL) is 10 times more likely to be injured than the radial collateral ligament.[21] Grade I and II injuries are when the ligament remains intact, whereas a grade III injury is a complete disruption of the UCL.

Mechanism of injury

UCL injuries occur from a forceful radial deviation of the thumb. This injury most frequently occurs in stick sports in which the thumb is abducted to hold a pole or stick, and then the athlete falls on an outstretched hand. Hence this injury is also referred to as "skier's thumb."[20,21]

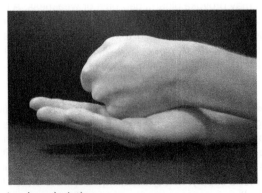

Fig. 4. Isometric wrist ulnar deviation.

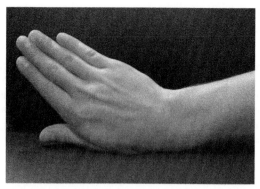

Fig. 5. Wrist ulnar deviation, when performed in neutral flexion and extension, exercises the ECU and flexor carpi ulnaris (FCU).

Evaluation findings

The athlete will report pain and tenderness at the ulnar side of the MCP joint. Weakness of pincer strength may be present. The injury is more likely to occur at the distal attachment, and an associated fracture at the base of the proximal phalanx occurs in about 50% of injuries.[20] A radiograph should be done to rule out such fractures before any manipulation of suspected UCL injuries. Failure to do so can turn a nonsurgical injury into one requiring surgery for an iatragenically displaced fracture. After ruling out fracture, MCP joint stability should be assessed with a radial stress at 30° of thumb flexion, to eliminate the false negative results often seen at 0° due to stabilization by the adductor aponeurosis.[12] Any significant discrepancy from the uninjured side is suggestive of injury. Most studies demonstrate at least a 15° difference in stability between sides, with greater than 35° being suggestive of a complete tear.[21–23] A stenar lesion occurs in a complete UCL tear, in which the proximal portion of the UCL displaces the adductor pollicis aponeurosis. The aponeurosis becomes interposed between the ligament and its insertion on the proximal phalanx and prevents healing, thus the need for surgical intervention.

Treatment

Nonoperative treatment is the preferred management for partial UCL injuries and non-displaced bony avulsions that are without lateral instability of the MCP.[20] Immobilization in a thumb spica cast typically lasts for 3 to 4 weeks, after which the athlete should have continued protection in a splint for 2 weeks. Discrepancies exist in the management of complete tears of the UCL and require consideration of the athlete's ability to function with the injury and while wearing a protective splint. Early operative intervention may afford the athlete the best surgical outcomes; however, studies also support the successful treatment of grade III injuries with 6 weeks of immobilization in a thumb spica cast.[13]

Rehabilitation of UCL injuries

Athletes can begin AROM that includes flexion and extension after casting is discontinued. Regardless of the course of treatment, care should be taken not to apply abduction stress to the MCP joint for the first 2 to 6 weeks after immobilization.[3] Once beyond the 8-week mark, athletes can also begin strengthening exercises, including work with putty.[3] Therapists need to be aware that thumb stiffness after immobilization is common with this injury. They should communicate with the treating physician about instituting the use of early active-motion protocols, which have been shown to be safe and effective (**Fig. 6**).[24]

RTP

If able to participate with a cast, RTP is allowed once the athlete is comfortable. If casting is not allowed, then RTP is dictated by the time it takes to be immobilized and regain ROM and near-normal strength. Special thermaplastic thumb spica splints that allow wrist motion can be fabricated for the athlete to wear during activity. Contact-sport athletes should have the thumb protected during sports for the remainder of the season.

Boxer's Fracture

Anatomy

A fracture of the metacarpal neck of the fifth finger is known as a boxer's fracture. The fifth metacarpal neck fracture is the most common fracture of the hand, because of the significant amount of movement of the fifth metacarpal.[12,13]

Mechanism of injury

A boxer's fracture occurs when there is direct impact against an object with a closed fist. The clenched fist position when punching is the most common mechanism.

Evaluation findings

Physical examination of a boxer's fracture will reveal swelling and tenderness on the dorsal aspect of the hand. The MCP joint may appear depressed, and malrotation of the fifth finger may also be present.[12] Because this type of fracture is often the result of a punching injury in a fight, inspection should be made for any evidence of an open wound. If skin integrity is compromised, evaluation for possible tooth fragments is necessary.

Three standard radiographic views of the hand are generally adequate to visualize the fracture. Because of the large amount of movement at the base of the fifth metacarpal with the carpus, surprising degrees of volar angulation are tolerated. However, if volar angulation of more than 40° is viewed on the radiograph, referral is necessary for possible open reduction.[11]

Treatment

Treatment of a boxer's fracture is immobilization in an ulnar gutter splint or a specialized thermoplastic splint that will immobilize only the MCP joints of the small and ring

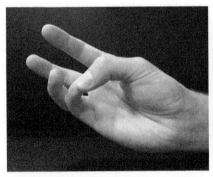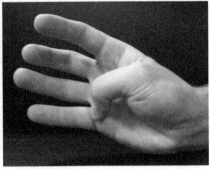

Fig. 6. Thumb ROM begins with opposition to each fingertip and progresses to flexion of thumb to base of each finger.

fingers, while allowing full IP and wrist ROM. Either splint should immobilize the fourth and fifth metacarpals with the MCP joints in 90° of flexion and the wrist in 30° of extension.[3] The splint is typically worn for 3 to 4 weeks. Generally, follow-up radiographs are done after 2 to 3 weeks to confirm stability of the fracture.

Rehabilitation of boxer's fractures

During immobilization, active and passive ROM should be maintained in all noninvolved joints. Once the splint is discontinued, active and passive ROM for the fourth and fifth MCP joints should begin. Gentle resistance exercises may begin as pain allows between weeks 4 and 6.[3] After 6 weeks, athletes can also begin light weightlifting activities with dumbbells and weight bars as tolerated.

RTP

If preliminary healing is present, and the athlete has no pain with movement, RTP in a protective playing cast is often allowed as early as 3 weeks.[13] Usually an athlete is allowed to play with only buddy tape by 6 weeks.[3]

Mallet Finger

Anatomy

The terminal extensor tendon is responsible for extension of the DIP. Mallet finger is caused by the avulsion of the extensor tendon from the dorsum of the base of the distal phalanx, with or without an avulsed fragment of bone.[25]

Mechanism of injury

Mallet finger typically results from forced flexion of the extended fingertip, caused by being struck by a baseball, softball, basketball, or volleyball.[26] However, mallet finger can also occur due to an extension axial load force.[2] The most frequently involved digits are the long, ring, and little fingers of the dominant hand.[25]

Evaluation findings

The patient with mallet finger will typically present with pain and inability to actively extend the affected DIP joint. Evaluation reveals a DIP that is swollen and bruised, and tender to palpation over the dorsum of the joint. In most cases, a 50 to 60° flexion deformity will be present at the DIP joint due to the complete avulsion of the extensor tendon. However, in cases of a partial tear of the extensor tendon, the patient may have weak active extension and a loss of 5 to 20° of extension.[12]

Mallet finger injuries sometimes require referral to orthopedic surgeons. Surgery is often performed on those fractures that involve more than 30% of the articular surface of the distal phalanx or have associated DIP joint subluxation.[12]

Treatment

There are many different techniques for the treatment of mallet finger, but most experts agree that the DIP should be splinted in full extension or slight hyperextension.[25] Care should be taken to avoid excessive extension, because the dorsal skin can be compromised vascularly. Three of the most common splints are the stack splint, the perforated thermoplastic splint, and the aluminum foam splint. Patients should understand the importance of not flexing the DIP, and should be instructed to have assistance when changing or retaping their splint.

Rehabilitation of mallet finger injuries

Nonsurgical management is the standard of care for most mallet finger injuries. Continuous splinting of the DIP should be maintained for 6 to 8 weeks, followed by 2 to 3 weeks of nighttime splinting.[12] It is important to keep the DIP joint extended at all times, even when changing the splint and bathing. If the DIP is accidentally flexed during treatment, a new full-length course (6–8 weeks) is recommended.[25] Compliance with continuous splinting should be evaluated regularly, as ongoing patient education on the importance of immobilization is vital to ensure optimal outcome of mallet finger injuries. During DIP immobilization, therapists should encourage PIP flexion, as its motion will not affect healing.[3]

RTP

Immediate sports participation is allowed if the athlete can play his or her sport with a splinted DIP joint. Otherwise, RTP will occur around 6 to 8 weeks after the injury.[13] Athletes who are returning to a sport that will put them at risk for reinjury should continue to wear a protective splint even after the initial 6- to 8-week treatment period.

Jersey Finger

Anatomy

The FDP originates in the upper forearm and divides into 4 tendons (1 to each finger) that insert on the palmar base of the distal phalanx. The FDP is superficial to the FDS, and the tendons of the FDP must pass through the FDS to insert on the distal phalanx of each finger. The ulnar 3 digits share a common muscle belly, and thus independent flexion of any finger with the others restrained in extension requires an intact FDS function to that finger. The FDP tendon's blood supply comes from 2 sources: (1) vinculae arising from the tenosynovium; and (2) nutrients from the synovial fluid of the flexor tendon sheath.[2]

Mechanism of injury

Jersey finger is caused by the avulsion of the FDP tendon from its insertion on the distal phalanx. It typically involves the ring finger, but can occur on any finger, and is usually caused by forceful passive extension of a flexed DIP joint while grasping a jersey.[2]

Evaluation findings

The patient with jersey finger will typically present with pain and inability to flex the DIP joint. Evaluation reveals localized tenderness, pain, and swelling at the site of injury. In addition to the localized symptoms, the patient may have symptoms along the course of the FDP tendon that extend down into the palm. These symptoms occur when the FDP tendon has retracted into the palm, resulting in a palpable tender mass in the palm.[27] The DIP joint should be tested in isolation by stabilizing the MCP and IP joints in extension and having the patient try to flex the distal tip of the finger.[28] Lateral and oblique radiographs may reveal an avulsion fracture on the volar aspect of the DIP joint at the FDP attachment site.[26]

All acute cases of jersey finger should be referred to an orthopedic surgeon at the earliest opportunity. Leddy and Packer[29] described 4 types of FDP avulsion: type 1 involves the FDP tendon retracting into the palm; type 2 involves the FDP tendon retracting to the level of the PIP; type 3 involves a large bone fragment avulsed with the FDP; and type 4 involves the tendon avulsed from the bone fragment and retracted into the palm.[29]

Treatment

Treatment will depend on the severity of tendon retraction. The literature suggests that types 1 and 4 should be repaired within 7 to 10 days of the initial injury because of disruption of the blood and nutrient supply to the tendon. For type 2 cases, early repair is still the treatment of choice. However, treatment may be delayed for 6 to 8 weeks depending on specific circumstances, such as an athlete in midseason who wants to finish the season. If this occurs, the athlete must be informed that delaying surgery may result in a less-than-optimal outcome, and further retraction of the tendon could occur during athletic activity. For type 3 injuries, the repair may be delayed because of the tendon being maintained in its sheath, but it is advisable to have the repair performed within the first 2 weeks.[2]

It is not uncommon for an athlete to present to the sports medicine physician with a chronic FDP tendon avulsion. In most of these cases, delayed primary repair is no longer an option for treatment. Management of chronic jersey finger includes benign neglect, a flexor tendon graft, or a DIP joint arthrodesis if the joint is unstable.[2] Most investigators recommend benign neglect, because functional impairment is typically minimal.[26]

Rehabilitation of jersey finger injuries

The injured finger should be splinted with the DIP and PIP joints in slight flexion until the patient has been seen by a surgeon. Rehabilitation after surgical repair of an FDP avulsion typically involves controlled motion while wearing a customized splint for 6 weeks. This treatment helps promotes tendon healing but also allows for tendon excursion. Caution must be taken if the athlete is doing "too well" with motion, as good tendon glide means there is less scar holding the repaired tendon together and, therefore, more risk of rerupture. The athlete should not be allowed to use the injured hand for anything, or extend the wrist or fingers without the splint on, or actively flex the fingers, as all can result in rerupture.[3] This injury benefits from the expertise of a hand therapist using specific protocols and with knowledge of sports medicine so that the athlete can be educated on the rationale for the exercises and the timeline.[3] Progressive ROM continues for 12 weeks, and strengthening exercises are begun around 10 to 12 weeks (**Fig. 7**).

RTP

It is typically 4 to 6 months before return to sports is allowed. A repaired tendon needs to be protected for between approximately 10 to 12 weeks, and longer for sports that may result in sudden unexpected forces to the injured finger. For athletes who participate in sports that do not involve the hand, RTP may be much earlier.[13] To do this, the athlete's hand must be taped into a tight fist and then casted in wrist flexion.[3] The risk of rerupture increases with early return.

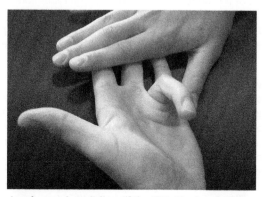

Fig. 7. Isolated exercises for tendon gliding of the FDS. The involved finger is allowed to flex and all uninvolved fingers are held in full extension.

Volar Plate Injuries

Anatomy
The volar plate forms the floor of the PIP joint and separates the joint space from the flexor tendons that pass superficially. The volar plate is comprises thick connective tissue, both ligamentous and cartilaginous in nature. Its main function is to prevent hyperextension of the PIP joint.[12]

Mechanism of injury
Volar plate injuries are caused by hyperextension of the PIP joint. They can occur in conjunction with dorsal subluxation, dislocation, or fracture-dislocation of the middle phalanx. In sports that require ball handling, hyperextension with axial loading is the most common cause of dorsal PIP dislocation.[2]

Evaluation findings
The patient with a volar plate injury presents with a painful and swollen PIP joint and a history of a hyperextension injury. Evaluation reveals pain and swelling, and increased tenderness on the volar side of the PIP joint. Ecchymosis may also be present on the volar side.

It is common to find a small avulsion fracture of the volar lip at the base of the middle phalanx on the radiograph. If a large (>40%), amount of the volar lip is fractured, a fracture-dislocation may be present and orthopedic opinion should be sought. It is important to assess joint congruity with these injuries. Parallel congruity should exist between the head of the proximal phalanx and the dorsal base of the middle phalanx. A "V" sign indicates joint subluxation.[30] Failure to diagnose joint subluxation with volar plate injuries is common and may result in serious complications.[12]

Treatment
Acute treatment of small, nondisplaced volar plate avulsion fractures consists of buddy taping or wearing a dorsal splint with the PIP joint in slight flexion. Treatment of large, displaced volar plate avulsion fractures consists of first reducing the dorsal subluxation of the middle phalanx. Closed reduction is preferable, but sometimes this is not possible and an open reduction must be performed. Treatments include immobilization in a dorsal extension block splint, closed reduction with percutaneous pin fixation for 10 to 14 days, followed by extension block splinting, and open reduction internal fixation if the fracture fragment is large enough.[2]

If a dorsal extension block splint is used, the PIP joint should initially be positioned equal to the amount of flexion required to maintain the reduction. This flexion is typically between 45 and 60°. The splint should be positioned so that active PIP flexion can be performed.[12] It is imperative that weekly radiographs be performed during the first 4 weeks after the initial injury to ensure that good alignment and reduction is maintained.[30]

Rehabilitation of volar plate injuries
With small nondisplaced volar plate avulsion fractures, buddy taping or splinting should be continued until the athlete is pain free. At 1 week postinjury, active ROM exercises should be started to avoid permanent stiffness and swelling of the PIP joint. Athletes should continue to buddy tape their injured finger during practice and competition for 6 to 8 weeks following their initial injury. Athletes should also be informed that some joint swelling can persist for 6 to 12 months after the injury.[12]

The primary goal of treatment of large displaced volar plate avulsion fractures is to restore joint stability.[30] This can be accomplished with nonsurgical and surgical interventions, depending on the stability of the joint. Most unstable PIP joints can be managed with an extension block splint that is worn for at least 4 weeks, and up to 8 weeks. The amount of PIP flexion is decreased by 10 to 15° each week until full extension is achieved. Throughout this time, the athlete should be encouraged to maintain flexion of the PIP and DIP joints.[12] Once full extension is achieved, the athlete should buddy tape the injured finger for 4 to 6 weeks while participating in athletic activities.

Regardless of whether the intervention is surgical or nonsurgical, the goal of treatment is to begin movement as soon as stability is evident. Rehabilitation should be individualized for each patient. However, it is usual to begin active ROM early, followed by active-assisted ROM and PROM once the fracture has healed. Strengthening exercises can be initiated when there is a solid union and full ROM is present.[30]

RTP
Depending on the sport, some athletes may be able to function while wearing an extension block splint, allowing RTP as soon as comfort allows. If this is not possible, athletes can return once they transition to buddy taping. Typically, athletes will continue with buddy taping for several weeks after the standard treatment period as a means to protect the joint during activities that may predispose them to reinjury.[12]

Central Slip Avulsion/Boutonniere Deformity

Anatomy
The central slip of the extensor tendon inserts into the base of the middle phalanx, resulting in an extensor force across the PIP joint. The lateral bands, formed by the lumbrical and interosseous tendons, travel on both sides of the proximal phalanx and pass dorsal to the PIP joint. The bands continue to course distally until they rejoin at the site of the triangular ligament on the middle phalanx and insert into the base of the distal phalanx, exerting an extensor force across the DIP joint.

Injury to the central slip can cause the lateral bands to retract and displace laterally and volarly, resulting in a flexed PIP joint and a hyperextended DIP joint, which is the classic boutonniere deformity.[26]

Mechanism of injury
A disruption of the central slip can be caused by direct trauma to the dorsum of the PIP joint, an acute flexion force at the PIP joint, or it can occur as a result of a volar dislocation of the PIP joint.[2] Injury typically occurs when an athlete receives a blow to the dorsum of the middle phalanx while actively extending the finger, which forces the PIP into flexion.[26]

Evaluation findings
The patient with a central slip injury will likely not demonstrate classic signs of a boutonniere deformity on initial evaluation. If left untreated, the boutonniere deformity will develop in the 4 to 6 weeks following the initial injury.[12] The athlete usually presents with a painful and swollen PIP joint and an inability to actively extend the PIP joint. It is important to distinguish a boutonniere deformity from the more typical "jammed" finger, which is caused by injury to the collateral ligaments. Boutonniere deformities will have maximal tenderness over the dorsum of the PIP joint and jammed fingers will be more tender on the sides of the joint.

Treatment
Acute boutonniere deformities should typically be splinted, with the PIP joint in full extension, with a dorsal padded aluminum splint. While splinted, the DIP and MCP should remain free for active and passive ROM exercises.[12]

Nonsurgical management is the standard of care for most boutonniere deformity injuries. Continuous splinting of the PIP joint in full extension should be maintained for 6 to 8 weeks, followed by night splinting for an additional 3 to 4 weeks.[12] It is recommended that splinting be maintained until full active PIP extension and full active DIP flexion is achieved.

Some boutonniere deformities should be referred to an orthopedic surgeon. Cases that involve a large displaced dorsal avulsion fracture may require surgical intervention.[12] Leddy and Packer[29] give 2 indications for repair of an acute central slip injury: (1) a PIP dislocation that cannot be reduced; and (2) a large displaced intraarticular PIP fracture at the base of the middle phalanx. Chronic boutonniere deformities may also require surgical intervention. However, Rettig[2] reports that most boutonniere deformities, acute and chronic, may be treated with conservative intervention consisting of splinting and an exercise program.

Chronic boutonniere deformities typically present with a flexion contracture. Serial casting or splinting in extension should be the first treatment for chronic injuries. If those treatments are unsuccessful, then surgical intervention to correct the contracture should be considered.[2]

Rehabilitation of boutonniere deformities

The athlete is splinted as discussed earlier, taking into account that, as the edema subsides, alterations to the splint will need to be made to avoid unnecessary motion at the PIP joint. Blocked PIP ROM exercises can be done to isolate flexion. Once the splint is removed, the athlete should progress through an ROM protocol, and then, at 10 to 12 weeks, strengthening of the grip can be added.[3]

RTP

Depending on the sport, some athletes will be able to return to practice and competition with their fingers braced or taped in extension.[2] Compliance with continuous splinting should be evaluated every 2 weeks during physician visits.

SUMMARY

Although the hand and wrist may be vulnerable to many different injuries during sports participation, a thorough evaluation and rehabilitation plan on the part of the sports medicine provider can speed the recovery process. By becoming comfortable with the anatomy and function of the hand and wrist, clinicians can enhance the ability of their athletes to return to full function after injury. Open communication between the physician and rehabilitation specialist will allow athletes to return to their sports in the safest and most time-efficient manner.

REFERENCES

1. Rettic AC, Ryan RO, Stone JA. Epidemiology of hand injuries in sports. In: Strickland JW, Rettig AC, editors. Hand injuries in athletes. Philadelphia: WB Saunders; 1992. p. 37–44.
2. Rettig AC. Athletic injuries of the wrist and hand. Am J Sports Med 2004;32: 262–73.
3. Schneider AM. Rehabilitation of wrist, hand, and finger injuries. In: Rehabilitation techniques for sports medicine and athletic training. 4th edition. New York: McGraw Hill; 2004. p. 452–84.
4. Rettig AC. Athletic injuries of the wrist and hand. Am J Sports Med 2003;31(6): 1038–48.

5. Pappas AM, Morgan WJ, Schultz LA, et al. Wrist kinematics during pitching. A preliminary report. Am J Sports Med 1995;23:312–5.
6. Rosenthal EA. The extensor tendons: anatomy and management. In: Hunter JM, Mackin EJ, Callahan AD, editors. Rehabilitation of the hand: surgery and therapy. 4th edition. St Louis (MO): Mosby; 1995. p. 519–84.
7. Hong E. Hand injuries in sports medicine. Prim Care 2005;32:91–103.
8. Ashe MC, McCauley T, Khan KM. Tendinopathies in the upper extremity: a paradigm shift. J Hand Ther 2004;17:329–34.
9. Forget N, Piotte F, Arsenault J, et al. Bilateral thumb's active range of motion and strength in de Quervain's disease: comparison with a normal sample. J Hand Ther 2008;21:276–85.
10. Walsh JJ. Fractures of the hand and carpal navicular bone in athletes. South Med J 2004;97(8):762–5.
11. Koval KJ, Zuckerman JD. Wrist. In: Handbook of fractures. 3rd edition. Philadelphia: Lippincott Williams & Wilkins; 2006. p. 237–56.
12. Eiff MP, Hatch RL, Calmbach WL. Carpal fractures. In: Fracture management for primary care. 2nd edition. Philadelphia: Saunders; 2003. p. 96–115.
13. Kovacic J, Bergfeld J. Return to play issues in upper extremity injuries. Clin J Sport Med 2005;15(6):448–52.
14. Grewal R, King GJ. An evidence-based approach to the management of acute scaphoid fractures. J Hand Surg Am 2009;34:732–4.
15. Jupiter JB. Current concepts review: fractures of the distal end of the radius. J Bone Joint Surg Am 1991;73A:461–9.
16. Jiuliano JA, Jupiter J. Distal radius fractures. In: Trumble TE, Budoff JE, Cornwall R, editors. Hand, elbow and shoulder: core knowledge in orthopedics. Philadelphia: Mosby Elsevier; 2006. p. 84–101.
17. Fernandez DL, Jupiter JB. Fractures of the distal radius: a practical approach to management. New York: Springer-Verlag; 1996.
18. Smith DW, Brou KE, Henry MH. Early active rehabilitation for operatively stabilized distal radius fractures. J Hand Ther 2004;17(1):43–9.
19. Glennon PE, Adams BD. Distal radioulnar joint and triangular fibrocartilage complex. In: Trumble TE, Budoff JE, Cornwall R, editors. Hand, elbow and shoulder: core knowledge in orthopedics. Philadelphia: Mosby Elsevier; 2006. p. 102–15.
20. Carlsen BT, Moran SL. Thumb trauma: Bennett fractures, Rolando fractures, and ulnar collateral ligament injuries. J Hand Surg Am 2009;34:945–52.
21. Taras JS, Hankins SM. Fractures and dislocations of the thumb. In: Trumble TE, Budoff JE, Cornwall R, editors. Hand, elbow and shoulder: core knowledge in orthopedics. Philadelphia: Mosby Elsevier; 2006. p. 56–68.
22. Heyman P, Gelberman RH, Duncan K, et al. Injuries of the ulnar collateral ligament of the thumb metacarpophalangeal joint. Biomechanical and prospective clinical studies on the usefulness of valgus stress testing. Clin Orthop Relat Res 1993;292:165–71.
23. Kuz JE, Husband JB, Tokar N, et al. Outcomes of avulsion fractures of the base of the proximal phalanx of the thumb treated nonsurgically. J Hand Surg Am 1999; 24:275–82.
24. Harley BJ, Werner FW, Green JK. A biomechanical modeling of injury, repair, and rehabilitation of ulnar collateral ligament injuries of the thumb. J Hand Surg Am 2004;29:915–20.
25. Bendre AA, Hartigan BJ, Kalainov DM. Mallet finger. J Am Acad Ortho Surg 2005; 13:336–44.

26. Peterson JJ, Bancroft LW. Injuries of the fingers and thumb in the athlete. Clin Sports Med 2006;25:527–42.
27. DeLee JC, Drez D. DeLee & Drez's orthopaedic sports medicine: principles and practice. Philadelphia: Elsevier Science; 2003.
28. Shippert BW. A "complex jersey finger": case report and literature review. Clin J Sport Med 2007;17:319–20.
29. Leddy JP, Packer JW. Avulsion of the profundus tendon insertion in athletes. J Hand Surg Am 1977;2:66–9.
30. Blazar PE, Steinberg DR. Fractures of the proximal interphalangeal joint. J Am Acad Orthop Surg 2000;8:383–90.

Rehabilitation of the Knee Following Sports Injury

Mark De Carlo, PT, DPT, MHA, SCS, ATC*, Brain Armstrong, MPT

KEYWORDS

• Knee • Rehabilitation • Sports • Conservative treatment

EPIDEMIOLOGY

Primary care physicians and other health care providers are often presented with various disorders related to the knee joint. Sports activities can subject the knee joint to severe stresses that increase the risk of both acute traumatic injuries and chronic overuse injuries. These disorders affect all generations from the elderly to the young athlete. Now more than ever children and adolescents are being pushed to the limits to succeed in their respective sport. More than 25 million students are involved in high school sports annually, and an estimated 30 million children in the United States participate in organized sports.[1] The knee joint is the second most commonly injured body site and the leading cause of high school sports–related surgeries.[2] An estimated 2.5 million adolescents visit emergency departments with sports-related injuries annually.[3] Children and adolescents are developing overuse syndromes and nontraumatic injuries due to intense training programs or participating in multiple sports in one season. At the college level, the knee joint is consistently among the most common sites of musculoskeletal injury, making up 20% to 36% of the total number of injuries encountered.[4] Due to recent technological advances, physicians are facing a population presenting with degenerative changes. Clayton and Court-Brown[5] came in contact with 1045 adult, soft tissue-related knee injuries over 5 years, which accounted for 37.4% of all adult soft tissue injuries presented.

The World Heath Organization in conjunction with the International Federation of Sports Medicine issues a consensus statement on organized sports for children. It is recommended that health professionals improve their knowledge and understanding of organized sports as well as risk and safety factors inherent to the sports participation.[6] This article is intended to provide primary care physicians and other

---

Methodist Sports Medicine Center/The Orthopaedic Specialists, 201 Pennsylvania Parkway, Suite 200, Indianapolis, IN 46280, USA
* Corresponding author.
E-mail address: mdecarlo@methodistsports.com (M. De Carlo).

Clin Sports Med 29 (2010) 81–106
doi:10.1016/j.csm.2009.09.004
0278-5919/09/$ – see front matter © 2010 Published by Elsevier Inc.

sportsmed.theclinics.com

health care providers with a better understanding of the importance of rehabilitation for these various knee injuries. As the number of athletes continues to grow and the number of knee injuries increases, patients will be looking for the most efficient and cost-effective treatment alternatives to provide them with an early return to play. Rehabilitation is a process that is designed to help athletes restore normal function following injury while providing interventions through an evidence-based approach on treating and preventing sport injuries. Through these various interventions athletes are provided an organized rehabilitation program that allows them to achieve optimal results in their respective sport.

CHILDREN AND ADOLESCENTS

Treating sports injuries in children and adolescents presents a unique challenge to the physician. Many times these individuals are seen for clinical conditions unique to their age group. Anterior knee pain is a frequent cause of complaint in young athletes.

Traction Apophysitis

Osgood-Schlatters (tibial apophysitis) is one of the most common knee problems in children between the ages of 10 and 15 years, and is seen in 13% of cases of knee pain in a typical sports medicine center.[7] These adolescents have undergone rapid growth and are involved in sports requiring repetitive quadriceps contraction, such as jumping and running. Repetitive overuse injury to the tibial tubercle apophysis causes this condition. The patient will present with intermittent aching pain that is made worse with participation in sporting activities, and is relieved by rest. Tenderness and an enlarged tibial tubercle region will present on examination. Pain with resisted knee extension and passive knee flexion is a common finding. The examination may also reveal poor flexibility of the quadriceps and hamstring muscle groups due to growth spurt. Thirty-five percent of patients with Osgood-Schlatters have symptoms in both knees.[8] Radiographs may reveal fragmentation and irregular ossification of the tibial tubercle.

Sinding-Larsen-Johansson is a condition similar to Osgood-Schlatters but instead of occurring over the tibial tuberosity, Sinding-Larsen-Johansson occurs at the inferior pole of the patella. Both conditions are overuse syndromes as the result of excessive activity or stress to the extensor mechanism. Typical clinical signs of Sinding-Larsen-Johansson are point tenderness a finger width above the inferior pole of the patella, and pain on sports participation, climbing stairs, and kneeling. Radiographs may show fragmentation or ossification of the inferior pole of the patella.

Management of these conditions is similar to that of the initial phase of rehabilitation, focusing on pain and inflammation control. Ice massage and iontophoresis are effective modalities to facilitate these goals. Avoidance of jumping, kicking, and running are essential to prevent stress to the extensor mechanism and promote healing. Phase II of rehabilitation addresses quadriceps and hamstring flexibility. The addition of eccentric strength training is an essential component in overcoming overuse injuries to the extensor mechanism.[9] Eccentric loading produces more stress on the patella tendon than concentric loading.[10] Exercises should be progressed bilaterally to unilaterally, with high repetition/low weight to low repetition/high weight. The rehabilitation progression is concluded with identification of training errors and recommendations to prevent further injury. A patella strap can be beneficial to control pain during sport activity.[11] Traction apophysitis is usually a self-limiting condition that allows sport-specific functional progression as tolerated.

Patella Tendinopathy (Jumper's Knee)

Patella tendinopathy is one of the most common overuse injuries involving the extensor mechanism. The condition is thought to result from repeated loading of the knee extensor mechanism, and is most prevalent in sports involving jumping.[12]

Terminology

A traditional term to describe this clinical condition is "patella tendinitis." Histopathological studies, however, have consistently shown the pathology underlying patellar tendinopathy to be degenerative rather than inflammatory.[12] The presence of the suffix "itis", implying the presence of inflammation, is often misused. "Tendinosis" is primarily used as a histopathological finding that is not correlated with clinical symptoms. The term "patellar tendinopathy", to be used in a clinical situation, in fact encompasses all clinical overuse conditions of the patella tendon, including those located at the proximal insertion at the inferior pole of the patella and those located at the distal insertion at the tibial tubercle or located at the main body of the patella tendon.[13]

Factors

The factors that contribute to the development of patella tendinopathy can be grouped into 2 categories: extrinsic and intrinsic. The most common extrinsic factor associated with patella tendinopathy is the repetitive overload of the extensor mechanism. This factor explains its prevalence in sports involving some form of jumping, such as basketball and volleyball. Intrinsic factors such as patella malalignment, patella alta, abnormal patellar laxity, and muscular tightness and imbalance have been determined to be causes of patella tendinopathy.[14] Johnson and colleagues[15] believe that impingement of the inferior pole against the patellar tendon during knee flexion contributes to the pathogenesis.

Diagnosis

The diagnosis can be made with a thorough history and clinical examination. Patients will present with well-localized anterior knee pain, which is exacerbated by activity, prolonged knee flexion, or ascending and descending stairs.[16] Patella tendinopathy typically presents with pain near the insertion of the tendon at the inferior pole of the patella. Pain will initially be present after sport activities. When the disease progresses, pain can be present during activity and can hinder an athlete's performance. Patients with chronic symptoms may exhibit wasting of the quadriceps, with the vastus medialis obliquus (VMO) portion most commonly effected.[17] An important differential diagnosis for patella tendinopathy is patellofemoral pain syndrome or Hoffa impingement. These conditions can coexist. A test used to differentiate between these conditions is to perform functional testing (decline squat), with or without tape, to influence the patellofemoral joint. Radiographs can be unremarkable but may reveal marked osteopenia in the distal pole of the patella.[18] The use of ultrasonography and magnetic resonance imaging (MRI) provides a detailed visualization of the tendon, which shows necrotic tissue (**Figs. 1** and **2**). Imaging should continue to be used as a supplemental aid to clinical examination and not a stand-alone tool in the assessment of patellar tendinopathy.

Conservative management is appropriate for overuse injuries to the extensor mechanism. As a consequence of the improved knowledge on the basic pathology of tendinosis, it has become evident that rehabilitation of the affected muscle-tendon unit should be the cornerstone of tendinopathy management. The time course of recovery with conservative management is equivalent to postoperative recovery and the

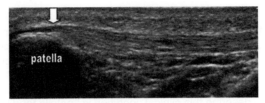

Fig. 1. Normal patellar tendon with its origin on the patellar inferior surface (*arrow*). Distal insertion not included on this longitudinal view. (*From* Brandon C, Lybrand M, Craig J, et al. Introduction to current concepts in musculoskeletal ultrasound: elbow, knee, and ankle. http://www.gehealthcare.com/usen/ultrasound/education/products/cme_msk.html. Accessed July 6, 2009; with permission.)

outcome of conservative management is equal to, if not better than, postoperative outcomes.[16] Development of a rehabilitation program should focus on unloading the tendon, promoting strength, and healing.

Initial conservative management should focus on patient education to reduce the loads applied to the extensor mechanism. The rehabilitation specialist should emphasize relative rest, correction of training errors and biomechanical faults, education on appropriate playing surface, flexibility, and strength. Relative rest rather than complete cessation of activity is appropriate. Relative rest is a partial reduction in the total amount or intensity of training hours. Correcting training errors and biomechanical faults can help to redistribute forces from the knee and patella tendon. Biomechanical correction during landing can be beneficial so that greater load is absorbed by the distal and proximal joints.[17] Also, a remarkable difference in incidence of patella tendinopathy exists depending on the surface played or trained on.[19] To assist in absorbing more load, correction of poor muscle flexibility through stretching exercises is beneficial. Proper flexibility of the quadriceps, hamstrings, iliotibial band, and calf muscles are necessary. Forces on the knee may also be influenced by foot mechanics, so correction should be made with foot orthoses if necessary. Appropriate loading is beneficial to tendon health, and strengthening exercises are recommended in the rehabilitation program. Strength exercises directed at the quadriceps and gluteal muscles are important in reducing the load on the patella tendon. Exercise prescription should focus on eccentric strengthening of the musculotendinous unit. Most research has supported the role of eccentric exercise in improving painful tendinopathy.[20–22] Eccentric programs have changed over time, but little evidence exists to suggest that one program has superior results to another. Purdam and Cook[23] suggested performing eccentric strengthening on a decline board. Their rationale was

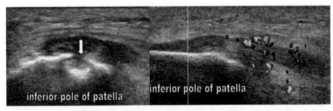

Fig. 2. Transverse (*left*) and longitudinal (*right*) views of jumper's knee with cortical irregularity of the distal patella. (*From* Brandon C, Lybrand M, Craig J, et al. Introduction to current concepts in musculoskeletal ultrasound: elbow, knee, and ankle. http://www.gehealthcare.com/usen/ultrasound/education/products/cme_msk.html. Accessed July 6, 2009; with permission.)

that passive and active calf tension has the capacity to reduce demand on the knee extensors in the squat by limiting forward angulation of the tibia. This angulation may be minimized by ensuring the calf functions at a shorter length, thereby developing less tension as the squat is performed. Several studies have confirmed that inclusion of eccentric decline squats as part of the rehabilitation program is essential (**Fig. 3**).[13,23–26]

The rehabilitation program must be progressive and logical, and each level must contain some form of eccentric strengthening. The rehabilitation program should begin with a strength-training bias, proceed with a power program, and conclude with sport-specific load exercises incorporating return to play.

Patella Instability

Patellofemoral pain syndrome (PFPS) is one of the most common knee disorders seen in orthopedic practice.[27] PFPS can be caused by a variety of factors, the most common of which is abnormal patellar tracking or patellar malalignment. PFPS typically affects younger people, 10 to 35 years old, and is more common in females than males.[10] Patella instability can be a difficult condition for clinicians to manage. McConnell[28] defines instability as the inability of the patella to stay within the confines of the trochlea from 20° of knee flexion. Differentiation needs to be made as to whether the problem is an acute injury, or recurrent instability. Predisposing risk factors contributing to patella instability include femoral anteversion, genu valgum, patellar or femoral dysplasia, patella alta, high Q-angle, pes planus, generalized laxity with genu recurvatum, overrelease of lateral retinaculum, previous patella dislocation, excessive external rotation of the tibia, and weakness of vastus medialis muscle relative to vastus lateralis.

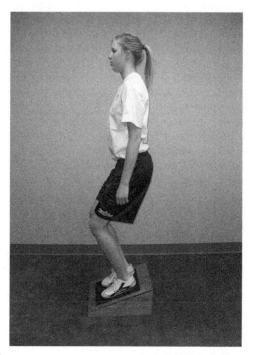

Fig. 3. Decline squat.

Diagnostic evaluation, such as radiographs, computed tomography (CT), or MRI, assists in the therapist's treatment plan. Radiographs should include 3 views of the patella, an anteroposterior (AP) weight-bearing view, a lateral view in 30° of flexion, and Merchant views. The AP view will reveal any fractures, and general presence of the patella can be viewed. The lateral view can show any patella alta or baja. The Merchant view may be the most important view, allowing the therapist to assess patellar tilt, patella subluxation, and trochlear dysplasia. A CT scan is effective in evaluating different malalignment patterns as well as assessing bone lesions and patellofemoral relationships. The CT scan is also valuable for diagnosis of recurrent patellar subluxation in adolescents. MRI is improving in its ability to detail osteochondral injury, and plays an important role in determining the location and extent of medial patellofemoral ligament (MPFL) injury.

The classic mechanism of acute injury includes a planting and cutting maneuver in which the femur rotates to promote knee valgus. At the same time, the quadriceps contracts pulling the patella superiorly, resulting in a lateral positioning of the patella and creating a force to displace the patella. The patella can also dislocate with contact, forcing the patella laterally. It is very rare for the patella to sublux or dislocate medially. The patient presents with complete loss of knee function, pain, and swelling, with the patella remaining in an abnormal lateral position. The patient with a chronically subluxing patella will present with pain as a result of swelling, but pain also results because the medial capsular tissue has been stretched and torn. Range of motion (ROM) will be restricted because of the resultant swelling.

Nonoperative management is sufficient for asymptomatic patients following first-time patella instability episodes. Rehabilitation of patellofemoral instability should concentrate on recruiting the VMO and gluteal activity, normalizing patellar mobility, increasing general flexibility and muscular control of the entire lower extremity, and addressing any other biomechanical problems that can be altered by treatment. Management varies between acute patellofemoral instability and chronic patellofemoral instability.

Following acute patella instability, it is imperative for the rehabilitation specialist to shorten the medial patellofemoral structures that have been disrupted. Phase I of rehabilitation following acute instability will require immediate cryotherapy with a brief period of immobilization. Swelling has a detrimental effect on quadriceps muscle activity, so the faster the swelling is reduced, the better the outcome for the patient.[29] The patient will most likely require a knee immobilizer with crutches for ambulation until full ROM and normal gait can be achieved. During gait the knee is often flexed so the normal heel/toe pattern in gait is lost, therefore gait training is emphasized early in the rehabilitation program. There are several patellofemoral braces claiming varying degrees of success in stabilizing the patellofemoral joint, which could be used for the acute dislocation.[30] Firm taping to shorten the medial retinacular tissue and MPFL providing stability for the disrupted tissue often allows a more normal gait pattern, and may improve the outcome of rehabilitation.[28]

Treatment of chronic instability will involve less drastic efforts to manage pain, inflammation, and effusion during phase I compared with acute instability. Patients with recurrent instability have hypermobile patellae, so the patella must be stabilized; this can be done with a patella-stabilizing brace or tape. Taping the patella can often determine if a brace will be effective in controlling excessive patellar motion. Patellofemoral pain syndrome is a difficult syndrome to manage in sports, due to the rehabilitation process and the need for patience on the part of the athlete. Patient education on this injury is critical during this phase.

Rehabilitation techniques in phase II are similar for both acute and chronic patella instability. The emphases of phase II is (1) regaining full ROM, (2) achieving dynamic patellar stabilization through quadriceps (VMO) and gluteal strengthening, (3) addressing lower extremity biomechanics, (4) normalizing patella mobility, and (5) improving soft tissue flexibility.

Although some clinicians believe it possible to isolate the VMO, there are no specific exercises that have been proven to isolate the muscle component. Therefore, when trying to strengthen the VMO, no specific exercise is better than another. Any knee extension exercise that elicits contraction of the VMO and does not cause pain is appropriate. **Figs. 4** and **5** show an individual performing short-arc knee extensions from 90° to 45°. There is increasing evidence that closed-chain training is more effective than open-chain exercises. Stensdotter and colleagues[31] found in asymptomatic subjects that closed-chain knee extension promoted a more simultaneous onset of electromyographic activity of the 4 different muscle portions of the quadriceps compared with open-chain knee extension. Escamilla and colleagues[32] reported a greater production of rectus femoris activity during open kinetic chain exercises, and closed-chain exercises produced more vastus activity. Closed-chain exercises allow additional strengthening of gluteal and trunk muscles as well. It has been found that 6 weeks of 1 session per week of physical therapy treatment changes the onset timing of VMO relative to vastus lateralis during stair stepping and postural perturbation tasks.[33]

Muscle stimulation may be used in conjunction with training as patients attempt to improve patella stability. Use of a biofeedback unit to monitor VMO contraction is a method that could be used to ensure VMO contraction. The biofeedback unit could also be used in conjunction with open- and closed-chain exercises. A randomized controlled trial that included specific weight-bearing gluteal and VMO training and also anterior hip structures stretches showed that the physical therapy group

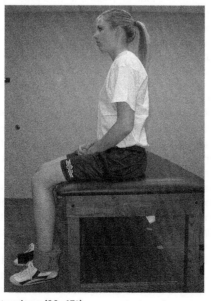

Fig. 4. Short-arc knee extensions (90–45°).

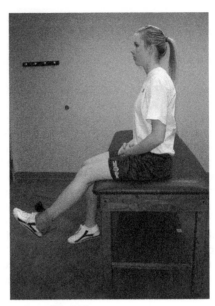

Fig. 5. Short-arc knee extensions (90–45°).

demonstrated a significantly better response to treatment and greater improvements in pain and functional activities than the placebo group.[34]

If lateral tracking of the patella is involved in the instability, correction of lower extremity biomechanics should be addressed. General conditioning and cross-training can be completed, such as aqua exercises and swimming. Key areas to evaluate and address during rehabilitation include gluteal strengthening, foot alignment, and flexibility of the rectus femoris, hamstrings, gastroc-soleus, and tensor fascia latae. Weakness of the gluteal muscles results in adduction and internal rotation of the femur during weight-bearing activities. Strengthening the gluteal muscles or taping the hip to promote external rotation of the femur will help address this problem. The most common problem that affects lower extremity alignment is excessive pronation of the subtalor joint that can lead to an increased Q-angle at the patellofemoral joint. Arch taping techniques, such as the Low-Dye technique, can be used to control pronation. If arch taping does not lessen symptoms, orthotics can be used with various medial forefoot posting.

Weber and Woodall[35] reported 3 common techniques to normalize patella mobility in patients who exhibit a laterally tracking patella due to tight lateral structures. The 3 most commonly reported techniques are manual patellar mobilization, patellar taping as described by McConnell, and iliotibial band/tensor fascia lata stretching. Kramer[36] reported success with manual lateral retinaculum stretching when it was used as part of a comprehensive patellofemoral rehabilitation program. He described 2 manual maneuvers: (1) medial patellar glide held for 1 minute with the knee extended to stretch the lateral retinaculum; and (2) patellar compression with tracking. McConnell[28] described taping techniques as a method to correct various malaligned patellar positions. She described 4 types of tape application: (1) correcting a lateral glide, (2) correcting a lateral tilt, (3) correcting an external rotation, and (4) correcting an anterior-posterior tilt, in which the inferior pole of the patella is tilted posterior. Patients must understand that taping is used as an adjunct to exercise and muscular balance, and not as a stand-alone tool. Taping is worn during activities that produce pain: just with athletics or with all activities of daily living. Once patella position is normalized, the patient is weaned from the tape. Finally, if during evaluation the iliotibial band and tensor fascia lata are found to be tight, stretching should be instituted.

With advance exercises and a functional progression, the athlete begins sports-specific activity with the use of a patella stabilization brace. An athlete is ready to return to his or her respective sport once patella position is normalized and the athlete passes a functional progression.

Plica Irritation

The medial patellar plica is the least common but most suspect to injury. The medial patellar plica is found in 20% to 60% of knees but does not necessarily cause symptoms.[37] This bandlike tissue can bowstring across the anterior aspect of the medial femoral condyle, impinging between the articular cartilage and the medial patellar facet during knee flexion. This action could cause anteromedial knee pain and snapping or clicking with pseudolocking, mimicking a patellofemoral or meniscal problem. Sports that require repetitive flexion-extension motion (eg, rowing, swimming, cycling) create microtraumas. Dupont[38] found that among symptomatic medial plicae in 98 patients, 81% were athletes: 18 runners, 11 cyclists, 9 swimmers, 9 horse riders, 8 gymnasts, and 8 dancers. Dupont[38] also found this syndrome most frequent in teenagers, when meniscal and ligamentous lesions are still rare. Inflammation to this tissue is usually caused by trauma or a twisting injury that results in synovitis. Medial patellar pain is the most constant symptom. Pain can be intermittent and is associated with repeated knee flexion/extension such as ascending and descending stairs, walking, and squatting. The painful arc occurs between 30° and 60° of flexion.

Common pathologies that imitate medial plica irritation include medial collateral ligament sprain, medial meniscal tear, and pes anserine bursitis. Also included in the differential diagnosis is degenerative joint disease, osteochondritis dissecans, and patellar malalignment. Most patients with plica irritation will have normal radiographs; however, it is important to rule out any bony pathology that could contribute to the irritation of the medial synovial plica. Ultrasonography enables dynamic examination of the plica. MRI has been found to be useful in the evaluation of thickness and extension of medial parapatellar plicae.[39]

If a medial plica syndrome is diagnosed, conservative treatment is always preferable initially, as it is cost-effective compared with arthroscopic surgery. Amatuzzi and colleagues[40] found conservative treatment to be effective in 60% of cases. Physical therapy focuses on using extensor mechanism rehabilitative techniques and inflammatory control to reverse tissue changes. Phase I of rehabilitation focuses on inflammatory control using phonophoresis and ice massage. Rest and avoidance of overuse activities, including sports, initially is recommended. Phase II consists of stretching and strengthening exercises to reduce compression over the anterior compartment of the knee. Stretching of the hamstrings, gastrocnemius, and quadriceps assists in decompressing the patellofemoral joint. Caution must be taken when performing open kinetic chain strengthening exercises in terminal extension to reduce irritation. Phase III consists of participation in sport/occupational-specific functional progressions.

ADULTS
Iliotibial Band Syndrome

Iliotibial band (IT band) syndrome is an inflammation of the IT band as it repeatedly moves across the lateral femoral condyle. As the knee moves from full extension to flexion, the IT band shifts from a position anterior to the lateral femoral epicondyle to a position posterior to the epicondyle. The transition occurs at about 30° of flexion. The repetitive flexion and extension of the knee in running or cycling can lead to irritation of the IT band as it passes back and forth over the lateral femoral epicondyle. IT band syndrome is the most common cause of lateral knee pain in runners, with a reported incidence as high as 22.2% of all lower extremity injuries.[41] The primary initial complaint in patients with IT band syndrome is diffuse pain over the lateral aspect of the knee. With time and continued activity, pain is localized over the lateral femoral epicondyle or the lateral tibial tubercle. The pain may radiate proximally or distally, and may begin after the completion of a run or several minutes into a run; however, the pain may increase enough that further running becomes impossible. Patients will often have pain when on stairs, running downhill, and sitting for long periods of time with the knee in a flexed position.[42] An abnormal vaulting gait with the knee extended may be observed.

Several factors have been associated with IT band syndrome, including excessive running in the same direction on a track, downhill running, a lack of running experience, abrupt increase in running distance or frequency, and running long distances.[41] MacMahon and colleagues (MacMahon JM, Chaudhari AM, Adriacchi TP. Biomechanical injury predictors for marathon runners: striding towards iliotibial band syndrome injury prevention. Hong Kong: International Society of Biomechanics; 2000. Unpublished [available at http://w4.ub.uni-konstanz.de/cpa/article/viewFile/2485/2333]) found strength deficits in the hip abductors to play a role in the development of IT band syndrome. Other potential causes include leg-length discrepancies, hyperpronation of the foot, a tight IT band, and tight hip adductors and dorsiflexors.

The differential diagnosis of lateral knee pain includes biceps femoris or popliteal tendinopathy, patellofemoral stress syndrome, primary myofascial pain, degenerative joint disease, lateral meniscal pathology, lateral collateral ligament sprain, superior tibiofibular joint sprain, stress fracture, and referred pain from lumbar spine. If the diagnosis is evident, routine imaging is rarely indicated; radiographic results are usually normal. Radiographs may reveal a prominent lateral femoral epicondyle that may increase the risk of impingement by jutting into the impingement zone, and may be an indication of chronic impingement.[43] MRI may be requested if there is doubt about the diagnosis and to exclude intra-articular problems. Patients with IT band syndrome may show a thickened IT band at the level of the lateral femoral epicondyle.

The goal of the initial acute treatment phase is to reduce local inflammation and promote healing with ice massage, iontophoresis, ultrasound, and anti-inflammatory medication. Also emphasized are a nonantalgic gait, full ROM, and activity modification. All running and other potentially exacerbating activity, such as cycling, should be avoided to reduce the repetitive stress at the lateral femoral condyle. In patients with chronic IT band syndrome, transverse friction massage can be useful to create a localized inflammation and promote collagen realignment. Once pain and inflammation are resolved, the subacute treatment phase can commence. Stretching exercises, with particular attention to the tensor fascia lata/IT band/hip flexor complex, can be started during this phase. Research has found greater lengthening of the IT band when an overhead arm extension is added to the standing IT band stretch. The patient could also move into a more transverse plane stretch by bending downward and diagonally, while reaching out and extending the arms with clasped hands (**Fig. 6**).[41] Myofascial restrictions along the lateral hip and thigh should be addressed. Combining this treatment with the use of a foam roller and performing isolated stretches for the tight muscles is particularly effective in releasing myofascial restrictions (**Fig. 7**).[43] Hip abduction strengthening exercises can begin once ROM and myofascial restrictions

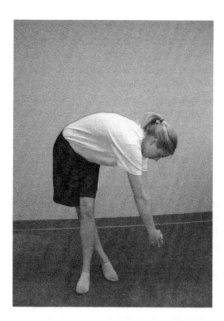

Fig. 6. IT band stretch.

are returned to normal. In patients with IT band syndrome, caution must be taken with exercise near terminal knee extension where the IT band passes over the lateral femoral condyle. It is initially recommended that one start with open-chain side-lying leg lifts, and then progress to closed-chain, single-leg balance step-downs and pelvic drop exercises. This approach enabled 22 of 24 injured runners to return to activities without symptoms or recurrence after 6 months.[44] Other closed-chain exercises such as squats, lunges, and leg press are beneficial in strengthening the hip abductors.

A running progression can begin only after the patient is able to perform all of the open- and closed-chain strengthening exercises with proper form and without pain.

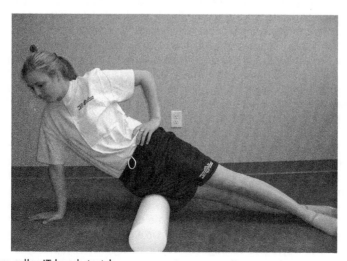

Fig. 7. Foam roller IT band stretch.

Abnormal foot mechanics should be addressed before beginning a functional progression to running. Orthoses may decrease the lateral knee stresses by controlling the foot's position. The return to running should be gradual, starting at an easy pace on a level surface. If the patient is able to tolerate this type of running without pain, mileage can be increased slowly. It is recommended that patients run every other day for the first week, avoiding any downhill running for the first few weeks. During the next 3 to 4 weeks, gradual increases in distance and frequency are permitted.

Osteoarthritis

Due to recent advances in medicine and the increasing population of older individuals, osteoarthritis has become a common condition presented to primary care physicians. The knee is a common site of osteoarthritis of the femorotibial and patellofemoral joints, possibly because it is often subject to trauma. Osteoarthritis usually begins in the medial or lateral tibiofemoral compartment, where it may be related to the articular cartilage damage that follows meniscal tears.[45] As the syndrome progresses, degenerative changes in either the lateral or medial compartment tend to increase the existing valgus or varus deformity. A varus deformity is the most common alteration of the osteoarthritic knee. This deformity results in increased forces on the medial compartment, which produces degenerative changes of the medial compartment, such as a degenerative medial meniscal tear. The varus deformity tends to cause abnormal gait mechanics, which produces patellofemoral arthritis and subsequent alteration of the extensor mechanism.

Whether the cause of osteoarthritis is idiopathic or posttraumatic, similar symptoms are presented. The major complaint is usually pain associated with effusion. Pain is aggravated by activity or weight-bearing activities but also can be aggravated at rest when one position is maintained for a long period of time. Morning stiffness that decreases with motion is a common complaint. The knee will become painful and stiff again if the patient exceeds the joint's limitations during prolonged standing or walking. Hertling and Kessler[45] describe a certain gait depending on which deformity is present. Lateral knee degeneration would result in a valgus knee, causing the knee to thrust medially during gait. Medial degeneration would result in a varus knee, causing the knee to thrust laterally during gait. The patient will present with quadriceps atrophy, which may be the result of a fixed flexion contracture. The end range of flexion and extension are also often limited, with joint stiffness.

Rehabilitation of osteoarthritis includes a variety of interventions, such as manual therapy techniques, balance, coordination, and functional retraining techniques, knee taping techniques, electrical stimulation, and foot orthotics. Rehabilitation specialists can address barriers that may prevent individuals with osteoarthritis from achieving maximum benefit from exercise or physical activity programs. Several investigators have published articles highlighting the beneficial effects of physical therapy in the outcome of osteoarthritis.[46–49]

Phase I of the rehabilitation program includes pain and inflammatory control, improving ROM, gait training, and patient education. Ice for swelling control and spasm relief, or heat application is beneficial in the chronic phase. Transcutaneous electrical nerve stimulation (TENS) helps to reduce or alleviate pain. One of the most common changes in the osteoarthritic knee is a knee flexion contracture, therefore patients should be taught early how to avoid contracture. Stretching of the hamstrings and gastrocnemius can prevent the detrimental effects of a knee flexion contracture. Manual therapy techniques assist in easing pain and decreasing stiffness to improve ROM. Deyle and colleagues[50] reported significant improvements in pain, the 6-minute walk test, and self-reported function scores in the manual therapy plus exercise group compared with the control group after 8 treatments delivered over 4 weeks. The patient's daily rituals need to be evaluated and adjusted accordingly. Simple active flexion and extension exercises should be done prior to weight-bearing activities. Walking is encouraged for daily activities but not in excess. Deep knee bends, sitting in low chairs, and remaining in the same position for prolonged periods should be avoided.

Phase II of the rehabilitation program includes exercises to strengthen the quadriceps, beginning with isometric exercises and increasing to progressive resistive exercises as tolerated. Full weight-bearing strengthening exercises should be used cautiously in the subacute and chronic phases, and avoided in the acute phase. Hydrotherapy has been shown to be as effective for unloading and weight bearing as closed kinetic chain exercises in the more acute phase.[51] In addition to exercises that improve strength, it is now being recommended that rehabilitation include balance and coordination, and provide patients with an opportunity to practice various skills that they will likely encounter during normal daily activities. These additional activities are believed to enhance confidence and skill in performing higher-level physical activity, which in turn may provide patients with appropriate tools for regulation participation in physical activity.[52] For individuals with patellofemoral arthritis, it has been recommended that patellofemoral taping techniques be used to supplement exercise for individuals to reduce pain during exercise and functional activities.[53] Biomechanical evaluation of the lower extremities and feet are recommended. Foot orthoses are occasionally used to indirectly offset faulty mechanics that may place harmful stress on the knee. Lateral wedge shoe inserts for individuals with medial compartment osteoarthritis are useful for reducing pain and improving function.

Phase III concludes with reintegration of normal daily activities and a daily exercise regime. The goals of phase III are to allow patients with knee osteoarthritis to return to higher levels of physical activity and maintain these levels of activity. Exercise, including a weight reduction program for patients who are obese, is a valuable treatment option for patients with pain and functional problems due to osteoarthritis of the knee.[47]

Meniscal Injuries

Injuries to the menisci are common in athletes. The sports with the highest incidence of meniscal injuries are soccer, football, basketball, and baseball. These sports require the athlete to perform planting, cutting, and rotational motions. The menisci move with the tibia in flexion-extension and with the femur during rotation. The medial meniscus has a much higher incidence of injury than the lateral meniscus, which may be attributed to being less mobile and its attachment to the medial collateral ligament. In cases of external rotation of the foot and lower leg in relation to the femur, the medial meniscus is most vulnerable. While in internal rotation, the lateral meniscus is most easily injured. Acute meniscus injuries are caused by a compression and twisting on a semiflexed knee. A contact mechanism is the result of a direct blow or force to the knee that causes a valgus, varus, or hyperextension force combined with rotation while the knee is in a weight-bearing position. Due to these forces, the meniscus becomes impinged within the tibiofemoral joint and tears. Noncontact mechanisms include a plant and cut maneuver or jumping. Again, athletes wearing cleats who are involved in contact sports are prone to meniscus injuries, occasionally in conjunction with ligament tears.

Lesions to the meniscus can be longitudinal, oblique, or transverse. A longitudinal tear of the anterior and posterior horns of the meniscus can produce a "bucket-handle" tear. The lateral portion slips over the dome of the medial femoral condyle and interferes with normal knee mechanics. This interference results in immediate locking of the knee joint so that the last 10° to 30° of extension is lost.

A meniscus tear often results in immediate joint-line pain with an effusion developing gradually over 48 to 72 hours. The person usually feels "a giving out" feeling with a deep pain. The torn meniscus may become displaced and wedge itself between the articulating surfaces of the tibia and femur, creating a "locking" or "catching" of the joint. A knee joint that is locked at 10° to 30° of flexion may indicate a tear of the medial meniscus, whereas a knee that is locked at 70° or more may indicate a tear of the posterior portion of the lateral meniscus.[54] Chronic meniscal lesions may also display recurrent swelling and obvious muscle atrophy around the knee. The patient may have complaints of an inability to perform a full squat or to change direction quickly when running without pain. The athlete may have a sense of the knee collapsing, or a "popping" sensation.

Not all meniscal tears will require surgery. Some meniscal tears may heal or become asymptomatic without surgical intervention. Rehabilitation varies depending on the course of treatment and type of meniscal injury. Nonoperative rehabilitation aims to reduce swelling, restore full ROM, normalize gait, and improve quadriceps function before returning to normal activities.

Phase I of meniscal injury rehabilitation focuses on controlling swelling and inflammation, increasing ROM, and normalizing gait. Cryotherapy is utilized to control pain and swelling. A compression garment can be used to assist in swelling control. The athlete should keep the leg elevated as much as possible following injury. If the meniscal injury is not a locked bucket-handle tear, regaining full extension is a critical factor in promotion of a normal gait and improvement in quadriceps function. The athlete may be partial weight bearing or weight bearing as tolerated, with the use of crutches, depending on the severity of the injury. Emphasis is placed on proper gait mechanics, focusing on extending the involved lower extremity landing on the heel and following through on the toe. The use of crutches can be discontinued once gait is normalized.

Phase II of the rehabilitation includes attaining full ROM, normal gait, no swelling, and improving quadriceps function. Low-impact cardiovascular workouts can begin, such as the stationary bicycle and stair stepper. Initial workouts should be 10 to 15 minutes in length and progress to 30 minutes with moderate to high resistance. Quadriceps-strengthening exercises are initiated to facilitate early return to normal strength. Once full ROM is regained and the athlete has sufficient leg control, weight room activities can begin. At the completion of this phase, light agility and sport-specific activities can commence.

Phase III of the rehabilitation focuses on a functional return to prior activity level. The athlete should be able to maintain full ROM and have no swelling. Strengthening should continue to focus on final sport-related deficits and limitations. Implementation of a sport-specific functional progression is appropriate at this time.

Ligamentous Injuries

Medial collateral ligament injury

Ligamentous injuries to the knee joint are very common in sports, and account for about 20% to 40% of all knee injuries sustained.[55] Sprains of the medial collateral ligament (MCL) occur regularly, and this is the most common injured ligament of the knee.[56] The MCL can tear at the midsubstance or either the femoral or tibial attachment sites. Approximately 65% of MCL sprains occur at the proximal insertion site on the femur.[54] Rehabilitation can vary substantially depending on the location of injury. MCL injuries occurring at the midsubstance or near femoral origin tend to develop stiffness and readily incur ROM loss. Restoration of full motion should be monitored closely within the first few weeks following injury. In contrast, injuries at the tibial attachment tend to heal with residual laxity and thus have easier return of ROM. As a result, additional protection may be required to allow the MCL to heal.[54] The MCL is most often injured as a result of a valgus force or combined valgus and external rotation forces. The MCL can be injured by an external force, such as a direct blow to the lateral aspect of the knee, common in football and hockey. In addition, this mechanism of injury can occur in a noncontact situation: a valgus force applied from a fall to the side with the ipsilateral leg kept firmly fixed. This type of injury is common in sports that involve cutting maneuvers such as soccer, basketball, and football.

The patient will present possibly with crutches, and the knee held in a slightly flexed position. Joint effusion will be present depending on the degree of injury, especially in the suprapatellar region. The patient will point to a localized area that corresponds well to the site of the tear as being the primary site of pain. If a moderately severe tear or complete rupture is present, the pain will largely subside as no fibers remain intact from which pain can arise. No effusion ensues because the capsule is usually torn, allowing the fluid to leak out of the joint cavity.

Since the early 1990s, the treatment of MCL sprains has changed considerably. The current approach is nonsurgical, and includes limited immobilization with early ROM and strengthening exercises. Shelbourne and Patel[57] found the best approach for management of a combined MCL/anterior cruciate ligament (ACL) injury was achieved by treating the MCL injury nonsurgically and performing a delayed reconstruction of the ACL. The results of several clinical studies have provided the basis for nonoperative treatment of MCL injuries.[57–61] These clinical studies have demonstrated excellent results using a treatment approach of immediate motion without surgical intervention for isolated MCL injuries. It is well accepted that isolated MCL injuries can heal with good stability and excellent functional results after nonoperative treatment. The optimal conditions for MCL healing are maintenance of the torn fibers in close continuity, an intact and stable ACL, immediate controlled motion, and protection of the MCL against valgus and external rotation stresses.[62]

The rehabilitation following an isolated MCL sprain can be broken down into 3 phases. Patient advancement will vary according to the location of the tear, degree of instability, concomitant injuries involved, age, and activity demands. Grade I injuries may be progressed as tolerated with or without the use of a hinged knee brace. Grade II injuries can be progressed as tolerated, depending on the patient's signs and symptoms. A hinged knee brace or immobilizer can be used early in the rehabilitation. Grade III injuries will be immobilized in 30° of flexion for 1 to 3 weeks. This protection provides a stable environment for proper healing and tightening of the injured ligament complex.

Phase I of the rehabilitation program involves initiation of ROM, promotion of early healing, and protection. Restoring ROM is progressed in a nonpainful arc of motion so the detrimental effects of immobilization can be prevented and collagen synthesis can be accelerated. The patient is encouraged to bear weight as tolerated with or without protective devices, to provide nourishment to the articular cartilage and subchondral bone. Cryotherapy is used as much as possible throughout the day to control pain and swelling. Immobilization is dependent on the patient's instability and pain. For patients with grade I MCL injury, bracing is used as needed. Patients with a grade II injury use a brace and possibly an immobilizer. Grade III injuries are managed with an immobilizer. The goals on completion of phase I are to minimize pain and swelling, and to attain full weight bearing and normal gait with or without a brace or immobilizer.

Phase II rehabilitation emphasizes restoring full nonpainful ROM and beginning a strengthening program for the entire involved lower extremity. Patients exhibit nearly full ROM, although terminal knee extension and flexion may still be limited because of pain. Patients should demonstrate a normal gait pattern with or without assistance from a hinged knee brace. Closed kinetic chain strengthening exercises are initiated to restore and enhance proprioception and neuromuscular control. Nonimpact aerobic training such as stationary bicycle, elliptical stepper, and stair stepper are employed. In addition, pool exercises may be initiated to improve total body conditioning and facilitate functional progression while limiting the stresses on the joint. On completion of phase II, the patient should possess full ROM and mild to no swelling.

The final phase of rehabilitation, phase III, focuses on return to functional activities. All exercises are progressed with particular focus on closed kinetic chain strengthening, endurance exercises, proprioception activities, and functional/agility drills. The goals of phase III include pain-free activities of daily living without a brace, weight room strengthening, completing a functional progression with a brace, and return to sport or work with a brace. A running program is initiated starting with jogging and progressing to sprinting, with an emphasis on drills and agility activities specific to the demands of the patient's lifestyle or sport. Successful completion of a functional progression constitutes the end of this phase. A functional knee brace may be used depending on the demands of the individual's activity or sport and degree if injury (**Fig. 8**). The patient will need to continue an exercise program to continually increase strength and function, not merely to maintain strength.

Lateral collateral ligament injury
The lateral aspect of the knee is well supported by secondary stabilizers and can be treated nonsurgically. Isolated injury to the lateral collateral ligament (LCL) is rare, and often is injured in combination with one of the cruciate ligaments or posterolateral joint capsule. When the secondary restraints, lateral capsule, and cruciate ligaments are torn, functional instability is common and surgical correction is usually required. LCL sprains result in a disruption at the fibular head either with or without an avulsion

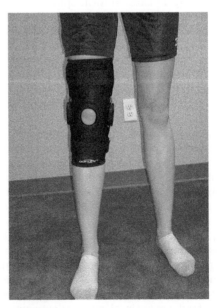

Fig. 8. Hinge knee brace.

in approximately 75% of the cases, with 20% occurring at the femur and only 5% as midsubstance tears.[63]

The mechanism of injury is usually hyperextension in combination with varus loading to the medial aspect of the knee. Patients will report they heard or felt a "pop" and there is immediate lateral pain. Swelling will occur rapidly and be extra-articular, with no joint effusion unless there is an associated meniscus or capsular injury.

The rehabilitation program following LCL sprains will follow the same progression as previously described for MCL sprains. Grade I injuries may be progressed as per patient tolerance with or without the use of a hinged knee brace. Grade II injuries can also be progressed as tolerated. A hinged knee brace can be used early in the rehabilitation, although an immobilizer may be used for patient comfort. Grade III injuries that are managed nonoperatively will be braced for 4 to 6 weeks, limited to 0° to 90° of motion.[54] Grade III LCL tears with associated ligament injuries that result in functional instability are usually managed by surgical repair or reconstruction.

Anterior cruciate ligament injury

Successful treatment options exist following ACL injury; however, an appropriate plan of care remains controversial. A more conservative approach may be appropriate for the sedentary individual in which the acute phase of injury progresses and then the individual participates in an organized rehabilitation program. These individuals are not involved in high-risk activities that include side-to-side twisting or jumping maneuvers. If the individual continues to have complaints of instability and difficulties with achieving normal function, then reconstructive surgery is considered. Most active and athletic patients prefer a more aggressive approach, and are willing to proceed with reconstructive surgery. Thus, successful surgical repair and reconstruction of the ACL-deficient knee is dependent on patient selection and their functional demands.

The most common mechanism of injury to the ACL includes a noncontact valgus and external rotation stress to the knee as the foot is planted on the ground. An isolated ACL injury can also occur with knee hyperextension with internal rotation. Combination injuries to the ACL, MCL, and the capsule can also occur with a valgus force and external rotation. Another combination injury of the ACL, LCL, and posterolateral capsule can occur with a varus force and internal rotation.

The patient will present with a swollen knee causing discomfort and pain. The swelling is usually a direct result of hemarthrosis. During history taking, the patient may recall a sudden pain or hear a "pop" followed by the knee giving way. The patient may with time develop a recurrent "giving way" problem due to instability. Active and passive ranges of motion are limited and painful.

Rehabilitation following ACL injury has changed dramatically over the past 30 years. Previous rehabilitation protocols resulted in complications including stiffness, weakness, and patellofemoral problems. **Tables 1** and **2** show a comparison of conservative and accelerated postoperative ACL rehabilitation. With the recognition of these complications, modifications in the pre- and postoperative rehabilitation program have been developed. An updated version of the accelerated rehabilitation program was first published in late 1990.[64] The accelerated rehabilitation is divided into 5 phases: phase I, preoperative; phase II, immediate postoperative; phase III, 2 to 4 weeks postoperative; phase IV, 4 to 8 weeks postoperative; and phase V, advanced rehabilitation and return to athletics. Progression from one phase to the next is based on the patients meeting goals outlined in each phase. The primary goals of ACL rehabilitation include restoration of knee stability, preservation of menisci and articular surfaces, and safe and expedient return to normal activities including athletics. This

Table 1
Conservative postoperative anterior cruciate ligament rehabilitation protocol

Time After Surgery	Exercises/Limitations
2–3 d	Casted at 30° of flexion Ab/adduction SLR Extension SLR Gluteal sets NWB ambulation with crutches
6–7 d	Discharged from hospital
2–4 wk	Cast removed, hinge brace applied at 30–60° ROM Passive ROM exercises Hamstring curls Ab/adduction and extension SLR Toe touch weight bearing
4 wk	Motion from 20° to 70° Add weights with SLR
8–10 wk	FWB as tolerated ROM 10–90° Passive stretching to increase ROM SLR with increased weight Eccentric knee extension Short-arc knee extension 90–45° Hamstring curls Bicycling, swimming
12–14 wk	ROM 0–110°, FWB Continue with previous exercises, start knee bends, step-ups, and calf raises
4 mo	ROM 0–120° Discontinue brace for ACL if good quad tone Increase intensity of exercise with higher weight and more sets and reps
6 mo	Isokinetic evaluation at 180°/s, 240°/s with 20° block Ligament stability test Jump rope, lateral shuffles Walking up to 2 miles Short arc to full knee extensions Squats, brace for activity
7 mo	Isokinetic evaluation Ligament stability test Quarter-mile walk/jog progression
8 mo	Agility drills including large figure-eights, lateral shuffles, backward running Isokinetic strengthening at slow and fast speeds Ligament stability test
9–12 mo	Return to normal activity levels if strength is greater than 80%, full ROM, no pain or swelling, and successful completion of functional progression

Summary of traditional postoperative ACL reconstruction rehabilitation protocol used from 1982 to 1986.

Abbreviations: ACL, anterior cruciate ligament; FWB, full weight bearing; NWB, non–weight bearing; ROM, range of motion; SLR, straight leg raises.

From DeCarlo M, Shelbourne KD, McCarroll JR. Traditional versus accelerated rehabilitation following ACL reconstruction: a one-year follow-up. J Orthop Sports Phys Ther 1992;15(6):309–16; with permission.

Table 2
Accelerated postoperative anterior cruciate ligament rehabilitation protocol

Time After Surgery	Exercises/Limitations
1–7 d	CPM and Cryo/Cuff Full passive hyperextension Increase flexion to 110° Obtain good leg control—SLR, active heel height WB as tolerated
1–2 d	Discharge from hospital
7–14 d	Terminal extension-prone hangs and towel extensions Increase flexion to 130°—wall slides, heel slides, active assisted flexion Progress from PWB to WB without crutches Achieve normal gait Increase leg strength—quarter-squats, calf raises Keep effusion to minimum
2–4 wk	Maintain hyperextension Regain terminal flexion Increase leg strength—weight room activities Bicycling and swimming Jump rope, single-leg hop, easy position drills
1–2 mo	Maintain full ROM Increase leg strength—single-leg strengthening Increase proprioception Isokinetic evaluation at 180°/s, 240°/s If greater than 70% start lateral shuffles, light sport-specific drills, cariocas, and jump rope Ligament stability test
3–6 mo	Full ROM Isokinetic evaluation Ligament stability test Continue weight room strengthening Return to sports if strength is greater than 80%, full ROM, no swelling, and successful completion of functional progression

Abbreviations: CPM, continuous passive motion; PWB, partial weight bearing; WB, weight bearing.
(Courtesy of Methodist Sports Medicine Center/The Orthopaedic Specialist, Indianapolis, IN.)

type of rehabilitation progression has been shown to demonstrate favorable outcomes among several clinicians.[64–70]

Phase I of the rehabilitation progression is the preoperative phase. The previous belief that there is an emergent need to reconstruct an acutely injured knee has been dispelled.[66] Instead of immediate surgery, the patient with an acutely torn ACL begins a rehabilitation program to prepare the injured knee and to ready him or her mentally for reconstructive surgery. The first component of phase I is focus on regaining full ROM, decreasing swelling, and resuming a normal gait pattern. It has been found that returning full symmetric knee ROM prior to surgery decreases complications such as arthrofibrosis.[71] Encouraging the patient to progress from partial to full weight bearing as tolerated stresses the importance of achieving a normal gait. Once swelling and pain are minimal and full knee motion is restored, strengthening exercises can begin. This phase allows the rehabilitation specialist the opportunity to educate the patient on the basic principles of the surgical procedure and postoperative rehabilitation expectations. The patient is ready for reconstructive surgery when the knee has no swelling, full ROM is present, and the patient fully understands the operative procedure and postoperative rehabilitation. Preoperative testing such as use of the KT-1000 knee ligament arthrometer, isokinetic strength evaluation, and single-leg hop test on noninvolved leg are all performed prior to surgery.

Phase II of the accelerated program includes the first 2 weeks after surgery. The goals of this phase are to (1) obtain full extension, (2) allow soft tissue healing, (3) maintain adequate quadriceps leg control, (4) minimize swelling, (5) achieve flexion of 130°, and (6) restore normal gait. Extension exercises are initiated immediately to minimize the potential problem of infrapatellar contracture, with the goal having equal hyperextension to the noninvolved knee. The patient is to remain lying down with the knee elevated in the continuous passive motion (CPM) device and ice throughout the first week to decrease swelling. Quadriceps control is initiated with exercises that emphasize active quadriceps contraction. Gait-training activities that involve heel-toe walking, retrowalking, and high-knee activities help restore normal gait. The combination of obtaining early extension and normal gait allows the patient to regain good quadriceps tone and leg control. This combination of clinical variables will set the pace for the entire rehabilitation program.

Phase III begins 2 weeks following surgery. Goals for this phase are full ROM and progression of strengthening exercises. During this phase patients are usually able to return to sedentary work, school, and activities of daily living. Aggressive ROM exercises are initiated to achieve full ROM. Functional strengthening is begun in this phase. Closed kinetic chain exercises are preferred for functional strengthening while open kinetic chain exercises facilitate isolated quadriceps muscle strengthening. High frequency and high repetitions are utilized to stimulate the patellar tendon graft harvest site.

Phase IV emphasizes advanced strengthening and the initiation of functional activities. If strength testing shows that the involved extremity has reached 70% of the strength of the unaffected leg, then a proprioceptive and light agility program can begin. A sport-specific functional progression can be developed toward the end of this phase. Agility training and restricted sports participation not only helps the patient regain quickness and functional movement patterns but also restores confidence in returning to previous functional status. Individual athletic drills should be sport specific. Throughout this phase, aggressive activity is progressed by the control of swelling and the maintenance of motion.

Phase V is the final phase of rehabilitation that includes progression of strengthening exercises and sport-specific drills with full return of activity. Strength and conditioning are adjusted according to the patient's specific needs. A functional progression is integrated to meet the patient's individual needs. Patients are counseled that although they can return safely as early as 2 months postoperatively, it takes an additional 3 to 4 months of sports-specific play for the patient to regain full confidence in his or her reconstructed knee.[68] Return to full, nonrestricted activities is the ultimate goal of the clinician and the patient for an optimal outcome.

Posterior cruciate ligament injury

Injury to the posterior cruciate ligament (PCL) in isolation is relatively uncommon in the athletic population. An athlete is much more likely to injure his or her ACL or MCL. The majority of PCL tears occur on the tibia (70%), whereas 15% occur on the femur and 15% are midsubstance tears.[63]

Rupture of the PCL is usually caused by a direct blow to the proximal tibia, a fall on the knee with the foot in a plantar-flexed position, or with hyperflexion of the knee. Less common causes include hyperextension or combined rotational forces. The injury may be isolated to the PCL, or associated with multiple ligament injuries or knee dislocation. Forced hyperextension will usually result in injury to both the ACL and PCL. If an anteromedial force is applied to a hyperextended knee, the posterolateral joint capsule may also be injured. Following PCL injury, the patient will indicate that they heard a "pop." Unlike ACL injuries, patients sustaining injury to the PCL will often believe that the injury was minor and that they can return to activity immediately. There will be mild to moderate swelling occurring within 2 to 6 hours.

Injury to the PCL results in changes in the kinematics of the knee. Changes in contact pressure can lead to degeneration of the medial tibiofemoral compartments and patellofemoral joint. The treatment of PCL injuries remains controversial. Isolated PCL injuries have been shown to do well with nonoperative treatment. Unlike a torn ACL and more like a torn MCL, the PCL may regain continuity with time. Shelbourne and colleagues[72] reported at follow-up, 63 of 68 patients with PCL injuries had the same or less clinical laxity than at their initial evaluations. The problem with PCL injury is not one of instability but rather one of progressive disability. Most studies demonstrate reasonably good functional outcomes after conservative treatment of isolated PCL injuries, yet a significant number of patients develop pain and early degenerative changes in the knee despite good functional recovery.[73]

In general, rehabilitation following PCL injury tends to be more conservative than after ACL injury, although follows a progression of rehabilitation similar to the progression of ACL rehabilitation. The severity of PCL injury will guide the aggressiveness of nonoperative therapy. Rehabilitation progression can be more rapid with grade I and II injuries, whereas grade III injuries are advanced more cautiously. Parolie and Bergfeld[74] reported a success rate of more than 80% with nonoperative treatment, and found that knee stability was not related to return to sport or patient satisfaction.

Phase I of the rehabilitation progression focuses on restoring full ROM, decreasing swelling and pain, and promoting normal gait mechanics. Unlike patients with ACL injury, most patients with an isolated PCL injury do not have extensive ROM limitations, quadriceps atrophy and weakness, or significant effusion. Due to passive motion placing minimal stress on the intact PCL, the use of a CPM device may be useful for grade III injuries treated nonoperatively. Patients with grade I and II injuries may begin passive ROM as tolerated. Weight bearing is encouraged in a range limited from 0° to 60° for mild injuries. Severe injuries require weight bearing to be completed in a brace locked in extension during the early treatment phase. A functional PCL brace may be used to prevent posterior displacement of the tibia from the effects of gravity and the weight of the leg, as well as the pull of the hamstrings.

Phase II continues with pain modulation, restoration of normal ROM and gait, and appropriate strengthening. Toward the end of phase I, the patient is encouraged to progress to full weight bearing without crutches. Once the patient is able to produce a normal gait pattern, the stance phase during normal gait is a basic form of closed kinetic chain quadriceps strengthening. By achieving this goal, the patient is able to regain good quadriceps tone and leg control, making it possible to include more challenging strengthening exercises. Working toward improving leg control and emphasizing normal gait are aimed at improving the patient's function. Quadriceps strengthening is the cornerstone of rehabilitation after PCL injury. The quadriceps function to dynamically stabilize the tibia and counteract the posterior pull of the hamstrings. Open kinetic chain activities may allow tremendous force to be exerted on the PCL during flexion exercises, therefore these exercises should be avoided initially. However, during open kinetic chain extension, minimal to no force appears to be generated in the PCL from 0° to 60°, as opposed to 60° to 90°, where significant stress is produced in the PCL.[73] Active closed kinetic chain activities of any kind, in any ROM, should be used cautiously when rehabilitating the PCL. If these exercises are used, they should be carried out in a ROM that limits flexion of the knee to about 45° or less to avoid generating higher forces in the PCL. The patellofemoral joint is at particular risk for the development symptoms during rehabilitation after PCL injury. Open kinetic chain extension exercises from 0° to 60° should be used very cautiously, due to the high joint reaction force across the patellofemoral joint.

Phase III includes return of full ROM and aggressive strengthening. The intensity of the current closed kinetic chain and open kinetic chain strengthening exercises may be increased, and isolated hamstring strengthening may be initiated at the end of this phase if needed. Low-impact cardiovascular exercises and swimming may also begin during this phase.

Phase IV of the rehabilitation progression includes restoration of normal flexibility and a gradual return to sports, with emphasis on return of power and endurance. The PCL brace may be removed if necessary. The closed kinetic chain and open kinetic chain strengthening programs can continue to advance, with the inclusion of isotonic hamstring strengthening if rendered appropriate. Running may begin in the pool, progressing to the treadmill and land as tolerated. Sport-specific functional progression such as agility drills and plyometric training should be included. Proprioceptive training needs to address static and dynamic balance deficiencies. The patient must safely pass an appropriate sport functional progression before returning to sports.

SUMMARY

Acquiring an injury to the knee can be devastating both physically and mentally. A rehabilitation specialist is necessary to allow the athlete to return to play at the optimal level. An effective rehabilitation program takes into consideration the anatomy of the involved structures, the biomechanics of the knee joint as well as the proximal and distal joints, the stage of healing, and the patient's response to treatment. Rehabilitation is done in a criterion-based progression that is based on individual progress from one phase to another and not over a prespecified period of time. If the rehabilitation deviates from this approach, the body will react with adverse affects such as inflammation, pain, and further injury. Delay in the entire rehabilitation program will delay the athlete in meeting goals and returning to play. Phase I focuses on restoration of ROM, pain modulation, inflammatory control, modification of activities, and gait training. Phase II is characterized by gaining full ROM, demonstration of normal gait pattern, basic to advanced strengthening and flexibility, appropriate cardiovascular conditioning, and proprioception retraining. Once the goals of phase II are accomplished, the patient can advance to phase III. Phase III allows functional return to prior activity levels. This phase includes a sport/occupational-specific functional progression. Appropriate taping, bracing, or protective devices may be needed as well. Utilizing the skills of a trained rehabilitation specialist will allow the athlete/individual an effective and efficient return to the prior level of function.

REFERENCES

1. Adirim T, Cheng T. Overview of injuries in the young athlete. Sports Med 2003; 33(1):75–81.
2. Ingram J, Fields S, Yard E, et al. Epidemiology of knee injuries among boys and girls in US high school athletics. Am J Sports Med 2008;36(6):1116–22.
3. Simon T, Bublitz C, Hambidge S. Emergency department visits among pediatric patients for sports-related injury. Pediatr Emerg Care 2006;22(5):309–15.

4. Bradley J, Honkamp N, Jost P, et al. Incidence and variance of knee injuries in elite college football players. Am J Orthop 2008;37(6):310–4.
5. Clayton R, Court-Brown C. The epidemiology of musculoskeletal tendinous and ligamentous injuries. Injury 2008;39:1338–44.
6. Lau L, Mahadev A, Hui J. Common lower limb sports-related overuse injuries in young athletes. Ann Acad Med Singapore 2008;37(4):315–9.
7. Peterson L, Renstrom P. Knee. Sports injuries—their prevention and treatment. 3rd edition. London: Martin Dunitz Ltd; 2001. p. 267–330.
8. Laor T, Wall E, Vu L. Physeal widening in the knee due to stress injury in child athletes. Am J Roentgenol 2006;186(5):1260–4.
9. Giffin R, Stanish W. Overuse tendonitis and rehabilitation. Can Fam Physician 1993;391762–9.
10. Fulkerson JP. Diagnosis and treatment of patients with patellofemoral pain. Am J Sports Med 2002;30(3):447–56.
11. Chew KTL, Lew HL, Date E, et al. Current evidence and clinical applications of therapeutic knee braces. Am J Phys Med Rehabil 2007;86(8):678–86.
12. Cook J, Khan K, Harcourt P, et al. Patellar tendon ultrasonography in asymptomatic active athletes reveals hypoechoic regions: a study of 320 tendons. Clin J Sport Med 1998;8(2):73–7.
13. Peers K, Lysens R. Patellar tendinopathy in athletes. Sports Med 2005;35(1): 71–87.
14. Witvrouw E, Bellemans J, Lysens R, et al. Intrinsic risk factors for the development of patellar tendinitis in an athletic population. Am J Sports Med 2001;29(2):190–5.
15. Johnson D, Wakeley C, Watt I. Magnetic resonance imaging of patellar tendonitis. J Bone Joint Surg Br 1996;78(3):452–7.
16. Khan K, Maffulli N, Coleman B, et al. Patellar tendinopathy: some aspects of basic science and clinical management. Br J Sports Med 1998;32(4):346–55.
17. Warden S, Brukner P. Patellar tendinopathy. Clin Sports Med 2003;22(4):743–59.
18. Pasque C, McGinnis D. The knee. In: Sullivan J, Anderson S, editors. Care of the young athlete. 1st edition. American Academy of Orthopedic Surgeons and American Academy of Pediatrics; 2001. p. 377–404.
19. Ferretti A. Epidemiology of jumper's knee. Sports Med 1986;3(4):289–95.
20. Bahr R, Fossan B, Loken S, et al. Surgical treatment compared with eccentric training for patellar tendinopathy (jumper's knee) a randomized, controlled trial. J Bone Joint Surg 2006;88(8):1689–98.
21. Visnes H, Bahr R. The evolution of eccentric training as treatment for patellar tendinopathy (jumper's knee): a critical review of exercise programmes. Br J Sports Med 2007;41(4):217–23.
22. Woodley B, Newsham-West R, Baxter G. Chronic tendinopathy: effectiveness of eccentric exercise. Br J Sports Med 2007;41(4):188–99.
23. Cook J, Purdam C. Rehabilitation of lower limb tendinopathies. Clin Sports Med 2003;22(4):777–89.
24. Frohm A, Saartok T, Halvorsen K, et al. Eccentric treatment for patellar tendinopathy: a prospective randomised short-term pilot study of two rehabilitation protocols. Br J Sports Med 2007;41(7):e7.
25. Jonsson P, Alfredson H. Superior results with eccentric compared to concentric quadriceps training in patients with jumper's knee: a prospective randomised study. Br J Sports Med 2005;39(11):847–50.
26. Young M, Cook J, Purdam C, et al. Eccentric decline squat protocol offers superior results at 12 months compared with traditional eccentric protocol for patellar tendinopathy in volleyball players. Br J Sports Med 2005;39(2):102–5.

27. Powers CM. The influence of altered lower-extremity kinematics on patellofemoral joint dysfunction: a theoretical perspective. J Orthop Sports Phys Ther 2003; 33(11):639–46.

28. McConnell J. Rehabilitation and nonoperative treatment of patellar instability. Sports Med Arthrosc 2007;15(2):95–104.

29. Spencer JD, Hayes KC, Alexander IJ. Knee joint effusion and quadriceps reflex inhibition in man. Arch Phys Med Rehabil 1984;65(4):171–7.

30. Shellock FG. Effect of a patella-stabilizing brace on lateral subluxation of the patella: assessment using kinematic MRI. Am J Knee Surg 2000;13(3):137–42.

31. Stensdotter A, Hodges P, Mellor R, et al. Quadriceps activation in closed and in open kinetic chain exercise. Med Sci Sports Exerc 2003;35(12): 2043–7.

32. Escamilla R, Fleisig G, Zheng N, et al. Biomechanics of the knee during closed kinetic chain and open kinetic chain exercises. Med Sci Sports Exerc 1998; 30(4):556–69.

33. Cowan S, Bennell K, Crossley K, et al. Physical therapy alters recruitment of the vasti in patellofemoral pain syndrome. Med Sci Sports Exerc 2002;34(12): 1879–85.

34. Crossley K, Bennell K, Green S, et al. Physical therapy for patellofemoral pain. Am J Sports Med 2002;30(6):857–65.

35. Weber M, Woodall W. Knee rehabilitation. In: Andrews J, Harrelson G, Wilk K, editors. Physical rehabilitation of the injured athlete. 3rd edition. Philadelphia: Saunders; 2004. p. 377–428.

36. Kramer PG. Patella malalignment syndrome: rationale to reduce excessive lateral pressure. J Orthop Sports Phys Ther 1986;8(6):301–9.

37. Kulund DK. The knee. The injured athlete. 2nd edition. Philadelphia: JB Lippincott; 1988. p. 435–512.

38. Dupont JY. Synovial plicae of the knee. Clin Sports Med 1997;16(1):87–122.

39. Sznajderman T, Smorgick Y, Lindner D, et al. Medial plica syndrome. Isr Med Assoc J 2008;11(1):54–7.

40. Amatuzzi M, Fazzi A, Varella MH. Pathologic synovial plica of the knee. Am J Sports Med 1990;18(5):466–9.

41. Fredericson M, Weir A. Practical management of iliotibial band friction syndrome in runners. Clin J Sport Med 2006;16(3):261–8.

42. Panni AS, Biedert R, Maffulli N, et al. Overuse injuries of the extensor mechanism in athletes. Clin Sports Med 2002;21(3):483–98.

43. Fredericson M, Wolf C. Iliotibial band syndrome in runners. Sports Med 2005; 35(5):451–9.

44. Fredericson M, Cookingham C, Chaudhari AM, et al. Hip abductor weakness in distance runners with iliotibial band syndrome. Clin J Sport Med 2000;10(3): 169–75.

45. Hertling D, Kessler R. Knee. Management of common musculoskeletal disorders—physical therapy principles and methods. 4th edition. Philadelphia: Lippincott Williams & Wilkins; 2006. p. 487–557.

46. Ettinger WH, Burns R, Messier SP, et al. A randomized trial comparing aerobic exercise and resistance exercise with a health education program in older adults with knee osteoarthritis. The Fitness Arthritis and Seniors Trial (FAST). JAMA 1997;277(1):25–31.

47. Jamtvedt G, Dahm KT, Christie A, et al. Physical therapy interventions for patients with osteoarthritis of the knee: an overview of systematic reviews. Phys Ther 2008; 88(1):123–36.

48. Rogind H, Bibow-Nielsen B, Jensen B, et al. The effects of a physical training program on patients with osteoarthritis of the knees. Arch Phys Med Rehabil 1998;79(11):1421–7.

49. van Baar ME, Dekker J, Oostendorp RA, et al. The effectiveness of exercise therapy in patients with osteoarthritis of the hip of knee: a randomized clinical trial. J Rheumatol 1998;25(12):2432–9.

50. Deyle G, Henderson N, Matekel R, et al. Effectiveness of manual physical therapy and exercise in osteoarthritis of the knee. Ann Intern Med 2000;132(3):173–81.

51. Woolfenden JT. Aquatic physical therapy approaches for the extremities. In: Cirullo JA, editor. Orthopaedic physical therapy clinic of North America. 3rd edition. New York: WB Saunders Company; 1994. p. 209–30.

52. Fitzgerald GK, Oatis C. Role of physical therapy in management of knee osteoarthritis. Curr Opin Rheumatol 2004;16(2):143–7.

53. Hinman R, Crossley K, McConnell J, et al. Efficacy of knee tape in the management of osteoarthritis of the knee: blinded randomised controlled trial. BMJ 2003; 327(7407):135.

54. De Carlo M, McDivitt R. Rehabilitation of the knee. In: Voight M, Hoogenboom B, Prentice W, editors. Musculoskeletal interventions: techniques for therapeutic exercise. New York: McGraw Hill; 2007. p. 607–50.

55. Powell J. 636,000 injuries annually in high school football. Athl Train 1987;2219–26.

56. Woo SL, Inoue M, McGurk-Burleson E, et al. Treatment of the medial collateral ligament injury II: structure and function of canine knees in response to differing treatment regimens. Am J Sports Med 1987;15(1):22–9.

57. Shelbourne KD, Patel DV. Management of combined injuries of the anterior cruciate and medial collateral ligaments. Instr Course Lect 1996;45275–80.

58. Hastings DE. The non-operative management of collateral ligament injuries of the knee joint. Clin Orthop Relat Res 1980;14722–8.

59. Sandberg R, Balkfors B, Nilsson B, et al. Operative versus non-operative treatment of recent injuries to the ligaments of the knee. A prospective randomized study. J Bone Joint Surg 1987;69(8):1120–6.

60. Shelbourne KD, Baele JR. Treatment of combined injuries of the anterior cruciate and medial collateral ligaments. J Bone Joint Surg 1988;156–8.

61. Wilk KE, Corzatt RD. In: Combined sections meeting of the American Physical Therapy Association; 1988.

62. Wilk KE, Andrews JR, Clancy WG. Nonoperative and postoperative rehabilitation of the collateral ligaments of the knee. Oper Tech Sports Med 1996;4192–201.

63. Tria A, Klein K. An illustrated guide to the knee. New York: Churchill Livingstone; 1991.

64. Shelbourne KD, Wilckens JH. Current concepts in anterior cruciate ligament rehabilitation. Orthop Rev 1990;19(11):957–64.

65. Fu F, Woo S, Irrgang J. Current concepts for rehabilitation following anterior cruciate ligament reconstruction. J Orthop Sports Phys Ther 1992;15(6):270–8.

66. Shelbourne KD, Wilckens JH, De Carlo M, et al. Arthrofibrosis in acute anterior cruciate ligament reconstruction. The effect of timing of reconstruction and rehabilitation. Am J Sports Med 1991;19(4):332–6.

67. Shelbourne KD, Nitz P. Accelerated rehabilitation after anterior cruciate ligament reconstruction. J Orthop Sports Phys Ther 1992;15(6):256–64.

68. Shelbourne KD, Klootwyk T, De Carlo M. Update on accelerated rehabilitation after anterior cruciate ligament reconstruction. J Orthop Sports Phys Ther 1992;15(6):303–8.

69. Shelbourne KD, Gray T. Anterior cruciate ligament reconstruction with autogenous patellar tendon graft followed by accelerated rehabilitation. A two- to nine-year followup. Am J Sports Med 1997;25(6):786–95.

70. Wilk KE, Andrews JR. Current concepts in the treatment of anterior cruciate ligament disruption. J Orthop Sports Phys Ther 1992;15(6):279–93.

71. Shelbourne KD, Patel DV, Martini DJ. Classification and management of arthrofibrosis of the knee after anterior cruciate ligament reconstruction. Am J Sports Med 1996;24(6):857–62.

72. Shelbourne KD, Davis TD, Patel DV. The natural history of acute, isolated, nonoperatively treated posterior cruciate ligament injuries. Am J Sports Med 1999; 27(3):276–83.

73. D'Amato M, Bach B. Knee injuries—posterior cruciate ligament injuries. In: Wilk KE, Brotzman B, editors. Clinical orthopaedic rehabilitation. 2nd edition. St Louis (MO): Mosby; 2003. p. 251–370.

74. Parolie JM, Bergfeld JA. Long-term results of nonoperative treatment of isolated posterior cruciate ligament injuries in the athlete. Am J Sports Med 1986;14(1): 35–8.

Rehabilitation of the Hip Following Sports Injury

Timothy F. Tyler, MS, PT, ATC[a,b,*], Aimee A. Slattery, MS, PT, CSCS[b,c]

KEYWORDS

- Hip • Linkage • Pelvic stability • Eccentrics
- Gluteus medius • Muscular slings

An athlete often presents to the rehabilitation specialist with either a nonspecific referral, such as "hip pain," or with a diagnosis of a more specific hip condition. It is the role of the rehabilitation specialist to look at movement above and below the injured site, to observe and evaluate global movement, such as sit to stand, and fine tuning and neuromuscular control of smaller, more specific supportive muscles. It is the rehabilitation specialist's job to take the athlete from a basic level of function to the highest level of sport activity. The rehabilitation specialist considers several key elements: boney structure, forces produced by myofascial properties, and neuromuscular control. The highly skilled clinician is trained to look at the "linkage" between the trunk and all parts of the lower extremity. Why is the hip not transferring the load well? Where is the breakdown? The gluteus medius (GM), pelvic stability, and supportive muscular slings are of great importance when optimizing the function of the hip. The hip is subjected to forces equal to multiples of the body weight and requires osseous, articular, and myofascial integrity for stability. This is the mind set when devising an athlete's rehabilitative program, looking at all influential factors that affect joint movement and integrity. Injuries to the hip can vary significantly depending on the specific sporting activity involved. Contact sports will have a higher incident of traumatic injuries such as fractures, contusions, and dislocations, whereas endurance sports like running, swimming, and biking can lead to abnormal stress patterns and overuse injuries. Regardless of the injury, proper diagnosis and intervention is the key to the athlete returning to their sport. The importance of maintaining open communication with the referring physician is of great value to the rehabilitation specialist. A referral of all pertinent diagnoses can help guide effective treatment. With greater specificity, the athlete's impairments can be addressed in a more timely and specific manner.

The occurrence of injuries to the hip, pelvis, and thigh is low compared with the other lower extremity regions.[1–5] Although statistically less prevalent, a pathologic

---

[a] NISMAT at Lenox Hill Hospital, 130 East 77th Street, New York, NY 10021, USA
[b] 2 Overhill road, Suite 315, Scarsdale, NY 10583, USA
[c] PRO Sports PT, Scarsdale, NY, USA
* Corresponding author. 2 Overhill Road, Suite 315, Scarsdale, NY 10583.
E-mail address: shoulderpt@yahoo.com (T.F. Tyler).

Clin Sports Med 29 (2010) 107–126
doi:10.1016/j.csm.2009.09.005
0278-5919/09/$ – see front matter © 2010 Elsevier Inc. All rights reserved.

condition of the hip can cause immediate gait abnormalities, lead to chronic pain and premature degeneration in the hip joint itself. These injuries can vary significantly depending on the specific sporting activity involved.[6] Contact sports have a higher incident of traumatic injuries such as fractures, contusions, and dislocations, whereas endurance sports such as running, swimming, and biking can lead to abnormal stress patterns and overuse injuries. Regardless of the injury, proper diagnosis and intervention is the key to the athlete returning to their sport.

THE REFERRAL

The cause of hip pain in the absence of trauma may be more difficult to determine.[7] Often a new patient presents to the clinic for an evaluation with a nonspecific referral titled "hip pain." With an abundant list of differential diagnosis, it is important to rule out nonmusculoskeletal causes of hip pain. Some of these causes include but are not limited to genitourinary problems, endometriosis, ovarian cyst, peripheral vascular disease, infectious disease, metabolic disease, and tumor.[7] It is beyond the scope of this article to discuss the path to differential diagnosis, but it is important for the physician to know that the rehabilitation specialist has broad medical knowledge and is trained to recognize "red flags." These red flags are signs and symptoms that are outside the scope of "normal" musculoskeletal pain or dysfunction related to the diagnosis given. The rehabilitation specialist's ability to adequately screen for conditions requiring further examination by a physician can lead to more timely treatment of serious medical conditions.[8] A recent example follows: a patient was referred for rehabilitation with a diagnosis of lumbar spine and left hip osteoarthritis with possible trochanteric bursitis. After the specialist's examination, significant findings were: pain severity out of proportion to the reported injury, the presence of night pain, a positive "sign of the buttock," and empty end feels of all hip joint motions, which represented a noncapsular pattern of joint restriction. The specialist determined the patient should return to his referring physician. A computerized tomography scan of the left hip revealed a metastatic lesion at the left proximal femur.[8] Some of the modalities used to treat pain, spasm, and inflammation, such as therapeutic ultrasound, are contraindicated in cases such as metabolic disease and cancer. The importance of maintaining open communication with the referring physician is of great value to the rehabilitation specialist.

The specific referral can be paramount when the patient has overlapping conditions. Often the athlete with an adductor strain can have trochanteric bursitis and possible athletic pubalgia. In these cases, a specific referral of all pertinent diagnoses can help guide effective treatment; rather than a referral of "hip pain;" with greater specificity, the athlete's impairments can be addressed in a more timely and specific manner.

THE ROLE OF PELVIC STABILITY

The primary function at the hip joint is to support the weight of the head, arm, and trunk, while also serving as the connection between the lower extremities and pelvic girdle. The hip is subjected to forces equal to multiples of the body weight and requires osseous, articular, and myofascial integrity for stability. The anatomic design of the hip is well suited to handle this task and the increased loads that can be transmitted during athletic competition.[9]

Muscle forces are required to press the sacrum between the hip bones, also called self-bracing. Without this, shear loading is not tolerated and there is disruption of load transfer to the hip joint creating a canvas of potential injury and dysfunction. This is especially true for the athlete, undergoing intense levels of shear and tensile force at a microscopic level. The role of pelvic stability and recruitment of supportive musculature is of vital importance to the hip.

How well load transfers to the lumbopelvic-hip region dictates how efficient function will be. This is the mind set when devising an athlete's rehabilitative program, looking at all influential factors that affect joint movement and integrity. The rehabilitation specialist considers several key elements: boney structure, forces produced by myofascial properties, and neuromuscular control. It is the rehabilitation specialist's job to take the athlete from a basic level of function to the highest level of sport activity.

It is the role of the rehabilitation specialist to look at movement above and below the injured site, to observe and evaluate global movement, such as sit to stand, and fine tuning and neuromuscular control of small specific supportive muscles, such as multifidus and transverse abdominus. There is evidence that activation of trunk and gluteal muscles is different in those with pain than those without pain. In 1 study, surface electromyographic activity was recorded from 7 trunk and hip muscles for the supporting leg during hip flexion in standing. Onset of muscle activity relative to initiation of the task was compared between groups and between limbs. The results showed onset of obliquus internus abdominus and multifidi occurred before initiation of weight transfer in the control subjects. Yet, the onset of these muscles and gluteus maximus was delayed on the symptomatic side and onset of biceps femoris was earlier in subjects with joint pain.[10] This suggests alteration in strategy for lumbopelvic stabilization that may disrupt load transference through the pelvis.

This concept is often seen in postoperative spine patients. Postoperative rehabilitation goes well until a return to a more progressive strength training program results in onset of new symptoms, such as trochanteric hip pain. The underlying cause is the inability to recruit deep multifidi, therefore proximal stability is compromised and distal mobility is impaired. The inability to stabilize the pelvis while performing dynamic lower extremity movement, such as a lunge, produces shear force to the spine, creating a compensatory strategy of gluteal activation, piriformis spasm, and undue stress on the hip joints. The acute and painful bursae can be treated with modalities, myofascial release to the involved soft-tissue structures, and ice to calm the area. In addition, the patients are given a series of progressive exercises to recruit deep sacral multifidi, transverse abdominus, and pelvic floor muscles. Together, multifidi and transverse abdominus (along with their fascia) form a corset of support for the lumbopelvic region. Without addressing the need for pelvic stability, proper load transference to the hips does not occur and hip discomfort persists.

Another nonspecific referral often seen in the clinic is "bilateral trochanteric bursitis." This is a hallmark sign for the rehabilitation specialist to evaluate what is going on above the hips. The spine, whether an inert structure or neuromuscular in nature, is almost always involved.

The concept of linkage is the premise that a muscle contraction produces a force that spreads beyond the origin and insertion of the active muscle. This force is transmitted to other muscles, tendons, fascia, ligaments, capsules, and bones that lie in series and in parallel to the active muscle. In this manner forces are produced quite distant from the origin of the initial muscle contraction. These integrated muscle systems produce slings of forces that assist in the transfer of load. There are 4 slings of muscle systems that stabilize the pelvis regionally, between the thorax and legs. The posterior oblique sling contains connections between the latissimus dorsi and the gluteus maximus through the thoracodorsal fascia (**Fig. 1**). The anterior oblique sling contains connections between the external oblique, the anterior abdominal fascia and the contralateral internal oblique abdominal muscle and the adductor of

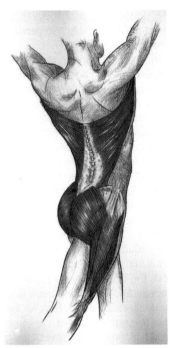

Fig. 1. The posterior sling provides pelvic stability through its connections with latissimus dorsi and gluteus maximus through the thoracolumbar fascia. (*From* Myers TW. Anatomy trains. Edinburgh: Churchill Livingstone; 2001; with permission.)

the thigh. The longitudinal sling connects the peroneii, the biceps femoris, the sacro-tuberous ligament, the deep lamina of the thoracodorsal fascia and the erector spinae. The lateral sling contains the primary stabilizers for the hip joint, namely the GM or gluteus minimus and tensor fascia latae, and the lateral stabilizers of the thoracopelvic region.

The movement specialist is responsible for returning the athlete to the highest level of performance. When addressing the hip, the clinician is responsible for making sure these slings are engaged and pelvic stability is solid (**Fig. 2**).

All too often the rehabilitation specialist examine the patient in the frontal and sagittal planes but fails to look at movement pattern in the transverse plane. More importance has been given to the patient's ability to control hip rotation during functional movements. In patients with patellofemoral pain syndrome, it has been suggested that a theoretic mechanism for pathology may be weak femoral external rotators that allow the femur to be in relative internal rotation and influence patellar alignment and kinematics. The role of the hip rotator muscles is frequently overlooked when addressing prevention and rehabilitation of knee and lumbar spine injuries. Weak and/or shortened hip rotators may contribute to abnormal lumbopelvic posture and cause compensatory motion in the lumbar spine during daily activities. The detrimental effects of inadequately conditioned and prepared hip rotators may predispose the athlete to lumbar spine injuries. The small external rotators of the hip (piriformis, obturator internus, obturator externus, gemellus superior, gemellus inferior, and quadratus femoris) sometimes get fatigued or overpowered by the large internal rotators of the hip (gluteus maximus, GM, and gluteus minimus) creating muscle imbalance.

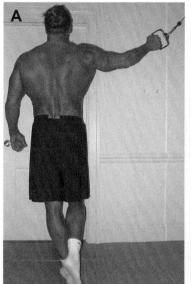 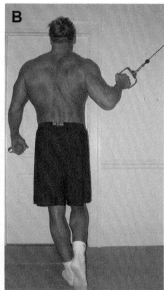

Fig. 2. (A) One-arm cable lateral pull with contralateral single limb stance: starting position. (1) Adjust the cable to slightly higher than the head. (2). The patient stands sideways with exercise arm closest to the pulley. (3) The patient grabs the pulley with 1 arm standing parallel to the cable column; upper extremity is in relative abduction. The patient is instructed to recruit and maintain engaged core muscles. (4) The patient then stands in single limb stance on the contralateral side. (B) Ending position. (1) The patient is asked to draw the scapula inward toward the spine first, then continue to perform a lateral pull. (2) The elbow should be drawn in as close to the trunk as possible, while keeping the upper arm within the frontal plane. (3) Good balance and posture should be maintained. (4) Note the posterior sling working together to create optimum pelvic stability.

A weak or dysfunctional GM has been linked to numerous injuries of the lower extremity and abnormalities in the gait cycle. The GM is responsible for preventing the opposite side of the pelvis from dropping during the stance phase of gait, commonly referred to as Trendelenburg gait, and plays a major role in providing frontal stability for the entire pelvis during walking and functional activities. The Trendelenburg gait has reduced gait efficiency and running speed; the athlete is at greater risk of developing lower back pain as a result of the pelvis not being stabilized during gait, jumping, and landing or when performing unilateral weight-training exercises.

A clinical pearl with regard to the GM is to manual muscle test each group of fibers to identify a more specific weakness. The anterior fibers, with connections to the tensor fasciae latae, are tested with the leg in abduction with femoral internal rotation (**Fig. 3**). The posterior fibers, with connections to the superior portion of the gluteus maximus, are tested with the leg in abduction with femoral external rotation. The posterior GM fibers, along with the gluteus maximus, contribute significantly to the vertical ground reaction force throughout the midstance phase of the gait cycle. The anterior fibers contribute little in the early stance phase of the gait cycle to support the hip, but then contribute greatly at the end of midstance. With assistance from joints and bones to gravity, the anterior and posterior medius/minimus generate nearly all the support evident in the midstance phase of the gait cycle.[11] One contributing factor to weak posterior fibers is the association with poor lumbopelvic posture.

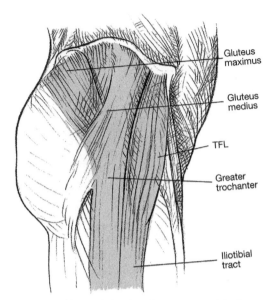

Fig. 3. Anterior and posterior fibers of the GM. (*From* Myers TW. Anatomy trains. Churchill Livingstone; 2001; with permission).

A patient in either an anterior pelvic tilt or posterior pelvic tilt has more difficulty recruiting the supportive musculature needed to maintain pelvic stability in the different phases of the gait cycle. In the running athlete, when the foot makes contact with the ground, the femur is in an abducted position in relation to the pelvis. Thus, the GM and tensor fascia latae are eccentrically loaded. As the running support phase progresses, these muscles must then contract as abduction at the hip occurs.[11] It is the role of the sports rehabilitation specialist to understand the biomechanical needs of the athlete, the timing, force, and recruitment patterns required of their task to achieve optimal performance from the musculoskeletal system.

An elementary exercise used to facilitate the posterior fibers of the GM is to have the patient prone with the knee flexed at 90°, isolate the GM with an isometric contraction (a manual cue is helpful), and then have the patient perform hip extension by lifting the thigh off the table. This position also inhibits the often contractured hip flexor muscle through reciprocal inhibition and aids in lengthening this muscle group; this facilitates better pelvic positioning and therefore improves the recruitment of the transversus abdominus and other core muscles. As timing and strength of the GM builds, progression of the exercise would move into more dynamic multiplanar functional training. As discussed with the runner, an eccentrically loaded GM may be targeted with a lateral step up exercise. A lateral rotational step up, as shown in **Fig. 4**, is a great functional exercise to isolate the posterior fibers of the GM and emphasize the transverse plane. Training the athlete to use the musculature as it would be used in sport-specific performance is the final goal.

GROIN PAIN

The evaluation and treatment of groin pain in athletes is challenging. The anatomy is complex, multiple pathologies often coexist, different pathologies may cause similar

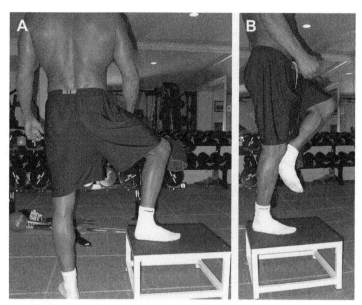

Fig. 4. (*A*) Facilitation exercise for GM posterior fibers: starting position: (1) The patient stands sideways parallel to the step. (2) The patient, without moving the position of the trunk, places the foot on the step in full hip external rotation. The foot will be at a 90° angle to the standing limb. (*B*) Ending position. (1) The patient is then asked to perform a step up. (2) The contralateral limb performs hip flexion to 90° to promote increased proprioception and dynamic balance. This limb is then placed back into the starting position on the floor. (3) The involved side with the foot in contact with the step is then placed back into starting position.

symptoms, and many systems can refer pain to the groin. Many athletes with groin pain have tried prolonged rest and various treatment regimens, and received differing opinions as to the cause of their pain.[12] The rehabilitation specialist is often given a nonspecific referral of "groin pain" or "anterior hip pain." The cause of pain could be as simple as the effects of a tight iliopsoas that requires stretching, or as complex as a sports hernia (SH).

An SH occurs when weakening of the muscles or tendons of the lower abdominal wall occur. This part of the abdomen is the same region where an inguinal hernia occurs, called the inguinal canal. When an inguinal hernia occurs, sufficient weakening of the abdominal wall exists to allow a pouch, the hernia, to be felt. In the case of an SH, the problem is caused by a weakening or tear in the abdominal wall muscles, but no palpable hernia exists.[13]

SH is a controversial cause of chronic groin pain in athletes. Most commonly seen in soccer and ice hockey players, SH can be encountered in various sports and in various age groups. Although there are several reports of SH in women, it is almost exclusively found in men. SH is largely a clinical diagnosis of exclusion. History of chronic groin pain that is nonresponsive to treatment should raise suspicion of SH, but physical examination findings are subtle and most diagnostic tests do not definitively confirm the diagnosis. Conservative treatment of SH does not often result in the resolution of symptoms. Surgical intervention results in pain-free return of full activities in most cases.[14]

The symptoms of SH are characterized by pain during sports movements, particularly twisting and turning during single limb stance. This pain usually radiates to the adductor muscle region and even the testicles, although it is often difficult for the patient to pinpoint. Following sport activity, the athlete is stiff and sore. The day after competition, mobility and practice is difficult. Any exertion that increases intraabdominal pressure, such as coughing or sneezing, can cause pain.[13]

A review based on the results of 308 operations for unexplained, chronic groin pain suspected to be caused by an imminent, but not demonstrable, inguinal hernia or an SH, were studied. No differences in perioperative findings between the cured and noncured athletes were found. It was characteristic that further clinical investigation of noncured operated athletes gave an alternative and treatable diagnosis in more than 80% of cases. Herniography was used consistently in the diagnostic process. In conclusion, the final diagnosis and treatment often reflects the specialty of the doctor and the present literature does not supply proper evidence for the theory that SH constitutes a credible explanation for chronic groin pain.[15] Nonoperative treatment usually involves a short period of rest followed by physical therapy focusing on abdominal strengthening, which may temporarily relieve the pain, but definitive treatment remains surgical repair and rehabilitation.[13]

A nonspecific referral of groin pain may be as serious as a labral tear. In a study of athletes undergoing arthroscopy, 60% were treated for an average of 7 months before it was recognized that the joint was the source of their problems. Most were initially diagnosed as various types of musculotendinous strains. Thus, it is prudent to include intraarticular pathology in the differential diagnosis when managing hip problems.[7] In a recent study, 90% of patients with a labral tear complained of groin pain. Direct MR arthrography is the best imaging modality for evaluation of underlying intraarticular disorders.[16] Researchers show a high positive predictive value of MR arthrography and higher sensitivity (90% and 91%) and accuracy (30% and 36%) compared with nonarthrogram MR images.[16] With increasingly sensitive MR imaging (MRI), today, a patient should not have to incur months of conservative treatment before realizing there is a chondral defect or a labral tear that must undergo hip arthroscopy to result in pain-free movement. The importance of open and professional communication between the physician and rehabilitation specialist is essential.

MUSCULAR STRAINS

Evaluation of hip bursitis, tendonitis, and muscle strains can be challenging when overlapping conditions exist. Certain exercises or specific stretches that stress the involved muscle can help determine which muscle is injured. In general, treatment and rehabilitation are designed to relieve pain, restore range of motion (ROM), and restore strength, in that order. Rest, ice, compression, elevation (RICE) is the standard protocol for mild to moderate muscle strains. Gentle massage to the area with ice helps to decrease swelling. Compression shorts or a wrap bandage may also be helpful in decreasing swelling and provide support. If walking causes pain, limited weight-bearing and crutches are considered for the first 1 or 2 days after the injury.

ADDUCTOR MUSCLE STRAINS

Adductor muscle strains can result in missed playing time for athletes in many sports, and are encountered more frequently in ice hockey and soccer.[17–19] These sports require a strong eccentric contraction of the adductor musculature during competition.[20,21] Recently, adductor muscle strength has been linked to the incidence of adductor muscle strains. Specifically, the strength ratio of the adduction to abduction muscles groups has been identified as a risk factor in professional ice hockey players.[22] Intervention programs can lower the incidence of adductor muscle strains but not avoid them altogether. Therefore, proper injury treatment and rehabilitation must be implemented to limit the amount of missed playing time and avoid surgical intervention.[23]

The main action of this muscle group is to adduct the thigh in the open kinetic chain and stabilize the lower extremity to perturbation in the closed kinetic chain. Each individual muscle can also provide assistance in femoral flexion and rotation.[24,25] The adductor longus is believed to be the most frequently injured adductor muscle.[26] Its lack of mechanical advantage may make it more susceptible to strain.

As discussed earlier, a thorough history and a physical examination is needed to differentiate groin strains from athletic pubalgia, osteitis pubis, hernia, hip-joint osteoarthrosis, rectal or testicular referred pain, piriformis syndrome, or the presence of a coexisting fracture of the pelvis or the lower extremities.

The exact incidence of adductor muscle strains in sport is unknown. This is due in part to athletes playing through minor groin pain and the injury going unreported. In addition, overlapping diagnosis can also skew the exact incidence. Groin strains are among the most common injuries seen in ice hockey players.[27–29] Groin strains accounted for 10% of all injuries in elite Swedish ice hockey players.[30] Furthermore, Molsa[31] reported that groin strains accounted for 43% of all muscles strains in elite Finish ice hockey players. Tyler and colleagues[22] published that the incidence of groin strains in a single National Hockey League (NHL) team was 3.2 strains per 1000 player-game exposures. In a larger study of 26 NHL teams, Emery and colleagues[18] reported that the incidence of adductor strains in the NHL has increased in the last 6 years. The rate of injury was greatest during the preseason compared with regular and post-season play. Prospective soccer studies in Scandinavia have reported a groin strain incidence between 10 and 18 injuries per 100 soccer players.[32] Ekstrand and Gillquist[19] documented 32 groin strains in 180 male soccer players representing 13% of all injuries in the course of 1 year. Adductor muscle strains, certainly, are not isolated to these 2 sports.

Previous studies have shown an association between strength and/or flexibility and musculoskeletal strains in various athletic populations.[19,33,34] Ekstrandt and Gillquist[19] reported that preseason hip abduction ROM was decreased in soccer players who subsequently sustained groin strains compared with uninjured players. This is in contrast to the data published on professional ice hockey players that found no relationship between passive or active abduction ROM (adductor flexibility) and adductor muscle strains.[22,35]

Adductor muscle strength has been associated with a subsequent muscle strain. Tyler and colleagues[22] found preseason hip adduction strength was 18% lower in NHL players who subsequently sustained groin strains compared with the uninjured players. The hip adduction to abduction strength ratio was also significantly different between the 2 groups. Adduction strength was 95% of abduction strength in the uninjured players but only 78% of abduction strength in the injured players. In addition, in the players who sustained a groin strain, the preseason adduction to abduction strength ratio was lower on the side that subsequently sustained a groin strain compared with the uninjured side. Adduction strength was 86% of abduction strength on the uninjured side but only 70% of abduction strength on the injured side. Conversely, another study on adductor strains on ice hockey players found no relationship between peak isometric adductor torque and the incidence of adductor strains.[35] Unlike the previous study, this study had multiple testers using a hand-held dynamometer, which would increase the variability and decrease the likelihood of finding strength differences. However, Emery and colleagues[35] showed that players who practiced during the off-season were less likely to sustain a groin injury as were rookies in the NHL. The final risk factor was the presence of a previous adductor strain. Tyler and colleagues[22] also linked pre-existing injury as a risk factor; in their study 4 of the 9 groin strains (44%) were recurrent injuries. This is consistent with the results of Seward and colleagues[36] who reported a 32% recurrence rate for groin strains in Australian Rules football.

Now that researchers can identify players at risk for a future adductor strain, the next step is to design an intervention program to address all risk factors. Tyler and colleagues[27] were able to show that a therapeutic intervention of strengthening the adductor muscle group could be an effective method for preventing adductor strains in professional ice hockey players. Before the 2000 and 2001 seasons, professional ice hockey players were strength tested. Thirty-three of these 58 players were classified as at risk, which was defined as having an adduction to abduction strength ratio of less than 80%, and placed on an intervention program. The intervention program consisted of strengthening and functional exercises to increase adductor strength (**Box 1**). The injuries were tracked over the course of the 2 seasons. In the present study there

---

Box 1
Adductor strain injury prevention program

Warm-up

    Bike

    Adductor stretching

    Sumo squats

    Side lunges

    Kneeling pelvic tilts

Strengthening program

    Ball squeezes (legs bent to legs straight)

        Different ball sizes

    Concentric adduction with weight against gravity

    Adduction in standing on cable column or elastic resistance

    Seated adduction machine

    Standing with involved foot on sliding board moving in sagittal plane

    Bilateral adduction on sliding board moving in frontal plane (ie, bilateral adduction simultaneously)

    Unilateral lunges with reciprocal arm movements

Sports-specific training

    On ice kneeling adductor pull togethers

    Standing resisted stride lengths on cable column to simulate skating

    Slide skating

    Cable column crossover pulls

Clinical goal

    Adduction strength at least 80% of the abduction strength.

were 3 adductor strains, all of which occurred in game situations. This gives an incidence of 0.71 adductor strains per 1000 player-game exposures. Adductor strains accounted for approximately 2% of all injuries. In contrast, there were 11 adductor strains and an incidence of 3.2 adductor strains per 1000 player-game exposures the previous 2 seasons before the intervention. In those previous 2 seasons, adductor strains accounted for approximately 8% of all injuries. This was also significantly lower than the incidence reported by Lorentzon and colleagues[30] who found adductor strains to be 10% of all injuries. Of the 3 players who sustained adductor strains, none of the players had sustained a previous adductor strain on the same side. One player had bilateral adductor strains at different times during the first season. These data show that a therapeutic intervention of strengthening the adductor muscle group can be an effective method for preventing adductor strains in professional ice hockey players.

Despite the identification of risk factors and strengthening intervention for ice hockey players, adductor strains continue to occur in all sports.[6] The high incidence of recurrent strains could be a result of incomplete rehabilitation or inadequate time for complete tissue repair. Holmich and colleagues[23] showed that a passive physical therapy program of massage, stretching, and modalities were ineffective in treating chronic groin strains. By contrast, an 8 to 12 week active strengthening program consisting of progressive resistive adduction and abduction exercises, balance training, abdominal strengthening, and skating movements on a slide board proved more effective in treating chronic groin strains. An increased emphasis on strengthening exercises may reduce the recurrence rate of groin strains. An adductor muscle strain injury program progressing the athlete through the phases of healing has been developed by Tyler and colleagues[27] and seems to be effective. As seen in **Box 2**, this type of treatment regime combines modalities and passive treatment immediately, followed by an active training program emphasizing eccentric resistive exercise. This method of rehabilitation program has been supported throughout the literature.[6]

HAMSTRING MUSCULAR STRAINS

The hamstrings are primarily fast-twitch muscles, responding to low repetitions and powerful movements. Hamstring muscle strains commonly result from a wide variety of sporting activities, particularly those requiring rapid acceleration and deceleration. An eccentric load to the muscle causes most of these injuries. Garrett and colleagues[37,38] showed that, in young athletes, hamstring muscle strains typically involve myotendinous disruption of the proximal biceps femoris muscle. Other investigators have also shown experimentally that the weak link of the muscle complex is the myotendinous junction.[37,39] Although apophyseal fractures of the ischial tuberosity have been reported in young athletes, most hamstring muscle strains are first and second degree strains.[40]

Hamstring muscle strains are among the most common injuries in sports involving high-speed movement and physical contact, and are by far the most commonly seen muscle strains in Australian Rules football with an incidence of 8.05 injuries per 1000 player-game hours. Soccer players are also susceptible to hamstring strains with an incidence of 3.0 per 1000 player-game hours for hamstring strains. Overall, any athlete who sprints as part of their sport may contribute to the incidence of hamstring strains.[36]

Factors causing hamstring muscle injury have been studied for many years. Age and previous injury were identified as the main risk factors for hamstring strain injury among elite football players from Iceland.[41] It has been suggested that muscle weakness, strength imbalance, lack of flexibility, fatigue, inadequate warm-up, and dyssynergic contraction may predispose an athlete to a hamstring strain.[42]

Fatigue has been implicated in the pathogenesis of muscle strain injury. Because muscle strains have been observed to occur either late in training or late in competitive matches, muscle fatigue has been indicated as a risk factor. Another study suggests that the injuries occur either early in games or training or late in games or training with

---

Box 2
Adductor strain post injury program

Phase 1 (acute)

   RICE for the first ~48 hours after injury

   Nonsteroidal antiinflammatory drugs (NSAIDs)

   Massage

   Transcutaneous electrical nerve stimulation (TENS)

   Ultrasound

   Submaximal isometric adduction with knees bent to with knees straight, progressing to maximal isometric adduction, pain free

   Hip passive range of motion (PROM) in pain-free range

   Non–weight-bearing hip progressive resistive exercises (PREs) without weight in antigravity position (all except abduction), pain-free, low load, high repetition exercise

   Upper body and trunk strengthening

   Contralateral lower extremity strengthening

   Flexibility program for noninvolved muscles

   Bilateral balance board

Clinical milestone

   Concentric adduction against gravity without pain

Phase 2 (subacute)

   Bicycling or swimming

   Sumo squats

   Single limb stance

   Concentric adduction with weight against gravity

   Standing with involved foot on sliding board moving in frontal plane

   Adduction in standing on cable column or Thera-Band (Hygenic Corporation, Akron, OH)

   Seated adduction machine

   Bilateral adduction on sliding board moving in frontal plane (ie, bilateral adduction simultaneously)

   Unilateral lunges (sagittal) with reciprocal arm movements

   Multiplane trunk tilting

   Balance board squats with throwbacks

   General flexibility program

Clinical milestone

   Involved lower extremity PROM equal to that of the uninvolved side and involved adductor strength at least 75% that of the ipsilateral abductors.

Phase 3 (sports-specific training)

    Phase 2 exercises with increase in load, intensity, speed, and volume

    Standing resisted stride lengths on cable column to simulate skating

    Slide board

    On ice kneeling adductor pull togethers

    Lunges (in all planes)

    Correct or modify ice skating technique

Clinical milestone

    Adduction strength at least 90% to 100% of the abduction strength and involved muscle strength equal to that of the contralateral side

---

inadequate warm-up and muscle fatigue, respectively, being the hypothesized reasons.[43] However, there are few quantitative data to support these statements. Croisier[44] has suggested that the persistence of muscle weakness and imbalance may lead to recurrent hamstring muscle injuries and pain. These investigators believe that when there is insufficient eccentric braking capacity of the hamstring muscles compared with the concentric motor action of the quadriceps muscles, the muscle may be at risk for injury.

Ekstrand and Gillquist[45] prospectively studied male Swedish soccer players and found hamstrings to be the muscle group most often injured. They noted that minor injuries increased the risk of having a more severe injury within 2 months. Others[46] have noted a recurrence rate of 25% for hamstring injuries in intercollegiate football players.

Most clinicians prescribe warm-up and stretching to help reduce the incidence of muscle strains. The evidence supporting this idea is weak and largely based on retrospective studies.[47] Following hamstring injury, the affected extremity and muscle group are significantly less flexible than the uninjured side, but there are no differences in isokinetic strength.[48] However, Jonhagen and colleagues[49] found decreased flexibility and lower eccentric hamstring torques in runners who sustained a hamstring strain compared with uninjured subjects matched for age and speed. The role of stretching and warm-up in injury prevention needs to be better understood so that optimal strategies can be developed.

There is no consensus for rehabilitation of the hamstring muscles after sustaining a strain. However, a rehabilitation program consisting of progressive agility and trunk stabilization exercises has been shown to be more effective than a program emphasizing isolated hamstring stretching and strengthening in promoting return to sports and preventing injury recurrence in athletes suffering an acute hamstring strain.[50] The aim of the physical therapy is to restore full pain-free ROM and strength throughout the ROM. In addition, as a complement to the usual restoration of function, the authors emphasize restoring eccentric muscle strength and correction of agonist/antagonist imbalances in the rehabilitation process. We recommend the inclusion of eccentric exercises at an elongated position of the hamstring muscles, submaximally, as soon as the patient can tolerate it. Our rationale is based on basic animal science research[51] and imaging studies of human muscle tissue[37] that have indicated incomplete healing following muscle strains. Fibrosis at the injury site is believed to be related to the risk of re-injury. Based on these observations, interventions aimed at remodeling the muscle tissue may be effective in reducing the risk associated with having had a prior muscle strain. Eccentric muscle contractions have been shown to result in muscle-tendon junction remodeling in an animal model,[52] and more recently have been shown to cause intramuscular collagen remodeling in humans.[53] Therefore, an eccentrically biased training program for previously injured muscles could theoretically reduce recurrence rates and would be worth studying in future research.

Rehabilitation would start with relative rest and protection of the injured muscle phase lasting from 1 to 3 days. Returning to exercise in this stage can lead to re-injury and disruption of the healing tissue. Multi-angle isometrics should be initiated to properly align the regenerating muscle fibers and limit the extent of connective tissue fibrosis. RICE, along with antiinflammatory medication, is helpful during the immediate stages of treatment. Heat, electrical stimulation, and ultrasound modalities can also be used in conjunction during the rehabilitation program to facilitate a return to competition. Heat is effective at increasing tissue temperature before stretching and exercise. Electric stimulation can be used to control edema and pain. Ultrasound is used as a deep-heating agent during the subacute phase to decrease spasm and prevent soft-tissue shortening. An effective strengthening program should treat the hamstrings as a 2-joint muscle and focus on concentric and eccentric contractions. Although lack of flexibility has been identified as a factor leading to hamstring injuries, the effectiveness of pre-exercise muscle stretching in reducing injuries has recently been questioned. In fact, recent studies cite decreased strength or power for up to 1 hour following passive stretching.[48] In theory, this decrease in force production is believed to result from the relaxation of the muscle-tendon unit. Therefore, before athletic competition, a general warm-up (jogging, cycling) to increase tissue temperature, followed by dynamic stretching that includes sports-specific movements is recommended. Examples of dynamic stretches for the legs include forward or backward lunges, high-knee marching and straight-leg kicks. Static stretching should be performed after the athletic activity.

LABRAL TEARS

Acetabular labral tears have become a commonly recognized source of intraarticular hip pain that affects athletes. Although strongly associated with athletes performing twisting pelvic motions and rotations of the hip that occur in sports such as soccer, golf, football, ballet, and hockey; athletes in all major sports (and even minor sports such as skateboarding and Olympic yachting) have been affected.[16] Isolated athletic injury or repetitive traumatic activity can lead to labral tears; however, underlying structural (femoroacetabular impingement) and developmental abnormalities predisposing athletes to labral lesions must be addressed. Recent studies have reported lesions associated with labral tears, and that labral tears rarely occur as isolated injuries. Return to sport is favorable in athletes who have labral tears if they are properly treated with arthroscopic intervention.[54] The incentive to return motivated athletes to a sport has proven fertile ground for advancement of arthroscopic techniques.[7] An emerging surgical trend, hip arthroscopy, is becoming more common, especially among athletes. The application of this minimally invasive technique, combined with advances in MRI, is considered a significant advancement in treating labral tears.

The hip is generally considered a statically stable joint because of large bony contact areas.[16] The femoral and acetabular surfaces correspond well to each other, but given the increased need for stability at this joint, an accessory structure is needed. The labrum not only deepens the socket, but increases the concavity of the socket through its triangular shape. This structural stability is reinforced by the hip joint capsule and its ligaments.

The onset of pain with an acute labral tear is immediate and usually located at the front of the hip joint. As with all hip problems, the pain may become diffuse and difficult to pinpoint. If the front of the hip joint is affected there may be a pinching sensation when the patient flexes the hip by bringing the knee up to the chest. A catching or giving way sensation in the hip may also occur. Symptoms usually occur when the hip is changing position. The pain may be reproduced in sport during activities that require concomitant weight-bearing and twisting (eg, driving a golf ball).[55]

Nonoperative treatment of labral tears can be successful if the tear is small and stable. The labrum (like the meniscus) has been shown to contain nerve endings (presumably related to nocioceptive and proprioreceptive function) and is believed to have low intrinsic healing ability because of low vascularity primarily obtained from the capsule.[7] If nonoperative means are not successful, the results of hip arthroscopy have been reported to have good results.[56] A return to sports is usually possible between 2 and 3 months after the operation.

Although the surgery is new and emerging, the rehabilitation progression should take into consideration the basic science principles of soft-tissue healing. As seen in **Box 3**, following surgery, the patient is instructed to use bilateral crutches with partial weight-bearing as tolerated for the first 2 weeks. Then, they are progressed to 1 crutch for 1 week, until they regain normal gait. Gait training to restore normal gait is paramount at this point in the rehabilitation. Some surgeons use a hip brace to restrict hip flexion ROM. During the second week the patient may also begin some easy pool walking and stationary biking without resistance. Independent ambulation is encouraged after 3 weeks. Aerobic activity is increased to 30 minutes along with active assistive hip ROM exercises. Any explosive movements or rotational hip torque could be potentially damaging to the hip capsule and labrum. For the first 4 to 6 weeks pain-free exercise is recommended to avoid a synovitis, tendonitis, or overstretch. At 2 weeks, light hip isotonics and more weight-bearing exercises such as bridges and single-leg bridges are initiated.

Strengthening of the hip extensors, abductors, and external rotators are emphasized along with light stretching for hamstrings, hip flexors, quadriceps, and the iliotibial band. The straight-leg exercise is avoided until the fourth week following surgery. Range of motion is pushed for internal rotation but progressed more slowly for external rotation. Trunk strengthening is begun at this time with emphasis on the transverse abdominus and the back extensors.

Six weeks after surgery, the patient begins light internal-external hip rotation stretching, the first time of stretching the postoperative hip beyond the active ROM. Eight weeks following surgery lower extremity strength work, which include squats, Romanian dead lifts, 4-way hip exercises, lunges, and lateral step work, is initiated. The lifting program, emphasizing lighter weights and higher repetitions, is designed to build endurance and avoid positions that could potentially aggravate the hip. It is important to avoid anything that causes either anterior or lateral impingement.

The rehabilitation specialist should be aware of any overlapping conditions such as low back pain and sacroiliac dysfunction. In addition, monitoring for the onset of flexor tendonitis and abductor tendonitis can help prevent failures. Patients with preoperative weakness in proximal hip musculature are at increased risk for postoperative tendonitis.[57]

Box 3
Arthroscopic hip labral repair rehabilitation guidelines

Weight-bearing status

    Foot flat with 20 lb of pressure

    Duration 2 to 4 weeks

Continuous passive motion

    Start 30 to 70°

    Increase as tolerated 0 to 90°

    Duration 2 weeks

Sleeping

    Ace wrap feet when sleeping for 2 weeks

Brace

    Daytime use

    Set at 0 to 90° of hip flexion

Stationary bicycle

    Immediate postoperation

    1 to 2 times daily for 15 to 20 minutes

    * Avoid pinching in front of hip by setting seat high

Pool exercises: begin on postoperative day 14 or as soon as sutures are removed and wound is healed

ROM

    Examination stool internal rotation: day 3 (may push early internal rotation within pain limits)

    Examination stool external rotation: day 7 (limit to 30° external rotation)

    2 to 3 sets of 12 to 15 repetitions

    Quadriceps rocking: day 7

    AROM: within limits of brace or as tolerated if no brace is worn

    PROM: within available pain-free limits after brace is removed

Strength

    Quad sets/ankle pumps: day 1

        Isometrics in neutral day 7 (*within painful limits)

        Bridges: day 7 to 10

        Isotonic weight equipment: day 14

            * Except for leg press, begin at 6 weeks

            * Shuttle or pilates, begin at 3 to 4 weeks dependent on weight-bearing

    Trunk strength

        * Transverse abdominus

        * Side supports

        * Trunk and low back stabilization as tolerated

Function

    No straight-leg raises for 4 weeks

May begin pool walking in chest high water

Avoid antalgic gait

Be aware of weakness of GM, side supports, and transverse abdominus strength in sagittal, coronal, and transverse planes

Balance

As soon as weight-bearing is permitted, begin working on double- and single-leg balance with eyes open and eyes closed

10 repetitions for 5 seconds is a good place to start

General considerations:

- Typically requires 3 months of supervised therapy
- Month 1: tissue healing phase (1–2 per week)

Goals:

Pain control

Decrease tissue inflammation

Decrease swelling

Maintenance of motion (flexion 0–90°; internal rotation as tolerated; external rotation 0–30°)

- Month 2: early functional recovery (2–3 per week)

Goals:

Full PROM

Progress to full AROM

Early strength gains

AVOID FLEXOR TENDONITIS AND ABDUCTOR TENDONITIS!

- Month 3: late functional recovery (2–3 per week)

Goals:

Advance strength gains, focus on abductor and hip flexor strength

Balance and proprioception

Continue to monitor for development of tendonitis

Progress to sport-specific activity in months 3 and 4 depending on strength

Do not progress to running until abductor strength is equal to contralateral side

Progression to sport-specific activities requires full strength and muscle coordination

Precautions:

- Avoid anything that causes either anterior or lateral impingement
- Be aware of low back or sacroiliac joint dysfunction
- Pay close attention for the onset of flexor tendonitis and abductor tendonitis
- Patients with preoperative weakness in proximal hip musculature are at increased risk for postoperative tendonitis
- Modification of activity with focus on decreasing inflammation takes precedence if tendonitis occurs

Following hip arthroscopy patients should avoid weight-bearing twists and turns on the hip for up to 3 months after surgery. Although not evidence-based, similar to a healing meniscus, this compression with rotation cannot be beneficial to a healing labrum in all age groups and all occupations. It is recommend that patients keep their movements within the midline, certainly for a 6-week period. They can then gradually introduce rotational movements to the hip, but such movements must be under their own control. Rotational therapeutic exercises should start with non–weight-bearing exercises and progress to full weight-bearing. After 3 to 4 months, assuming all is well, patients are allowed to return to unprotected, full activities provided full strength and coordination have returned.

SUMMARY

The rehabilitation specialist is often given the diagnosis of a specific hip condition. With the use of modalities and manual techniques, pain can be reduced and function restored. However, the highly skilled clinician is trained to look at the "linkage" between the trunk and all parts of the lower extremity. So much of the hip has to do with the quality of energy transfer: concentric versus eccentric, pronation (collapsing of the limb) versus supination (ability to reabsorb the energy that is transmitted through ground reaction forces). These questions are most significant when looking at injuries that are cumulative over time. Thus, when restoring normal pain-free function is difficult, the areas above and below the hip joint can provide the answers.

REFERENCES

1. Berend KR, Vail TP. Hip arthroscopy in the adolescent and pediatric athlete. Clin Sports Med 2001;20(4):763–78.
2. Byrd JW, Jones KS. Hip arthroscopy in athletes. Clin Sports Med 2001;20(4): 749–61.
3. Culpepper MI, Niemann KM. High school football injuries in Birmingham, Alabama. South Med J 1983;76(7):873–5, 878.
4. Gomez E, DeLee JC, Farney WC. Incidence of injury in Texas girls' high school basketball. Am J Sports Med 1996;24:684–7.
5. DeLee JC, Farney WC. Incidence of injury in Texas high school football. Am J Sports Med 1992;20:575–80.
6. Anderson K, Strickland SM, Warren R. Hip and groin injuries in athletes. Am J Sports Med 2001;29(4):521–33.
7. Thomas Byrd JW. The role of hip arthroscopy in the athletic hip. Clin Sports Med 2006;25(2):255–78 viii.
8. Van Wye WR. Patient screening by a physical therapist for nonmusculoskeletal hip pain. Phys Ther 2009;89(3):248–56.
9. Norkin L, LeVange P. Joint structure and function. Philadelphia: F.A. Davis Co; 1983.
10. Hungerford B, Gilleard W, Hodges P. Evidence of altered lumbopelvic muscle recruitment in the presence of sacroiliac joint pain. Spine 2003;28(14):1593–600.
11. Torry MR, Schenker ML, Martin HD, et al. Neuromuscular hip biomechanics and pathology in the athlete. Clin Sports Med 2006;25(2):187.
12. Harmon KG. Evaluation of groin pain in athletes. Curr Sports Med Rep 2007;6(6): 354–61.
13. Tyler TF, Nicholas SJ. Rehabilitation of extra-articular sources of hip pain in athletes. North Am J Sports Phys Ther 2007;2(4):207–16.
14. Moeller JL. Sportsman's hernia. Curr Sports Med Rep 2007;6(2):111–4.

15. Fredberg U, Kissmeyer-Nielsen P. The sportsman's hernia-fact or fiction. Scand J Med Sci Sports 1996;6(4):201–4.
16. Armfield DR, Towers JD, Robertson DD. Radiographic and MR imaging of the athletic hip. Clin Sports Med 2006;25(2):212–40.
17. Lynch SA, Renstrom PA. Groin injuries in sport: treatment strategies. Sports Med 1999;28(2):137–44.
18. Emery CA, Meeuwisse WH, Powell JW. Groin and abdominal strain injuries in the National Hockey League. Clin J Sport Med 1999;9:151–6.
19. Ekstrand J, Gillquist J. The avoidability of soccer injuries. Int J Sports Med 1983; 4:124–8.
20. Sim FH, Chao EY. Injury potential in modern ice hockey. Am J Sports Med 1978; 6(6):378–84.
21. Tegner Y, Lorentzon R. Ice hockey injuries: incidence, nature and causes. Br J Sports Med 1991;25(2):87–9.
22. Tyler TF, Nicholas SJ, Campbell RJ, et al. The association of hip strength and flexibility on the incidence of groin strains in professional ice hockey players. Am J Sports Med 2001;29(2):124–8.
23. Holmich P, Uhrskou P, Ulnits L, et al. Effectiveness of active physical training as treatment for long-standing adductor-related groin pain in athletes: randomized trial. Lancet 1999;353:339–43.
24. Moore KL. Clinically oriented anatomy. 3rd edition. Baltimore(MD): Williams & Wilkins; 1992.
25. Kendall FP, McCreary EK. Muscles: testing and function. 3rd edition. Baltimore (MD): Williams & Wilkins; 1983.
26. Renstrom P, Peterson L. Groin injuries in athletes. Br J Sports Med 1980;14:30–6.
27. Tyler TF, Campbell R, Nicholas SJ, et al. The effectiveness of a preseason exercise program on the prevention of groin strains in professional ice hockey players. Am J Sports Med 2002;30(5):680–3.
28. Jorgenson U, Schmidt-Olsen S. The epidemiology of ice hockey injuries. Br J Sports Med 1986;20(1):7–9.
29. Sim FH, Simonet WT, Malton JM, et al. Ice hockey injuries. Am J Sports Med 1987; 15(1):30–40.
30. Lorentzon R, Wedren H, Pietila T. Incidences, nature, and causes of ice hockey injuries: a three year prospective study of a Swedish elite ice hockey team. Am J Sports Med 1988;16:392–6.
31. Molsa J, Airaksinen O, Nasman O, et al. Ice hockey injuries in Finland. A prospective epidemiologic study. Am J Sports Med 1997;25(4):495–9.
32. Nielsen A, Yde J. Epidemiology and traumatology of injuries in soccer. Am J Sports Med 1989;17:803–7.
33. Knapik JJ, Bauman CL, Jones BH, et al. Preseason strength and flexibility imbalances associated with athletic injuries in female athletes collegiate athletes. Am J Sports Med 1991;19(1):76–81.
34. Orchard J, Marsden J, Lord S, et al. Preseason hamstring muscle weakness associated with hamstring muscle injury in Australian footballers. Am J Sports Med 1997;25(1):495–9.
35. Emery CA, Meeuwisse WH. Risk factors for groin injuries in hockey. Med Sci Sports Exerc 2001;33(9):1423–33.
36. Seward H, Orchard J, Hazard H. Collinson: football injuries in Australia at the elite level. Med J Aust 1993;159:298–301.
37. Speer KP, Lohnes J, Garrett WE. Radiographic imaging of muscle strain injury. Am J Sports Med 1993;21(1):89–96.

38. Garrett WE Jr. Muscle strain injuries: clinical and basic aspects. Med Sci Sports Exerc 1990;22:436–43.
39. De Smet AA, Best TM. MR imaging of the distribution and location of acute hamstring injuries in athletes. Am J Roentgenol 2000;174:393–9.
40. Wootton JR, Cross MJ, Holt KW. Avulsion of the ischial apophysis. The case for open reduction and internal fixation. J Bone Joint Surg Br 1990;72:625–7.
41. Arnason A, Sigurdsson SB, Gudmundsson A, et al. Risk factors for injuries in football. Am J Sports Med 2004;32(1):5–16.
42. Verrall GM, Slavotinek JP, Barnes PG, et al. Clinical risk factors for hamstring muscle strain injury: a prospective study with correlation of injury by magnetic resonance imaging. Br J Sports Med 2001;35(6):435–9.
43. Baumhauer JF, Alosa DM, Renstrom AF, et al. A prospective study of ankle injury risk factors. Am J Sports Med 1995;23:564–70.
44. Croisier JL. Factors associated with recurrent hamstring injuries. Sports Med 2004;34(10):681–95.
45. Ekstrand J, Gillquist J. Soccer injuries and their mechanisms: a prospective study. Med Sci Sports Exerc 1983;15(3):267–70.
46. Heiser TM, Weber J, Sullivan G, et al. Prophylaxis and management of hamstring muscle injuries in intercollegiate football players. Am J Sports Med 1984;12(5):368–70.
47. Dadebo B, White J, George KP. A survey of flexibility training protocols and hamstring strains in professional football clubs in England. Br J Sports Med 2004;38(4):388–94.
48. Worrell TW, Smith TL, Winegardner J. Effect of hamstring stretching on hamstring muscle performance. J Orthop Sports Phys Ther 1994;20(3):154–9.
49. Jonhagen S, Nemeth G, Eriksson E. Hamstring injuries in sprinters. The role of concentric and eccentric hamstring muscle strength and flexibility. Am J Sports Med 2005;22(3):262–6.
50. Sherry MA, Best TM. A comparison of 2 rehabilitation programs in the treatment of acute hamstring strains. J Orthop Sports Phys Ther 2004;34(3):116–25.
51. Nikolau P, Macdonald B, Glisson R, et al. Biomechanical and histological evaluation of muscle after controlled strain injury. Am J Sports Med 1987;15(1):9–14.
52. Frenette J, Cote CH. Modulation of structural protein content of the myotendinous junction following eccentric contractions. Int J Sports Med 2000;21(5):313–20.
53. Mackey A, Donnelly A, Turpeenniemi-Hujanen T, et al. Skeletal muscle collagen content in humans following high force eccentric contractions. J Appl Physiol 2004;97(1):197–203.
54. Bharam S. Labral tears, extra-articular injuries, and hip arthoscopy in the athlete. Clin Sports Med 2006;25(2):279–92, ix.
55. Byrd JW, Jones KS. Diagnostic accuracy of clinical assessment, magnetic resonance imaging, magnetic resonance arthrography, and intra-articular injection in hip arthroscopy patients. Am J Sports Med 2004;32(7):1668–74.
56. Byrd JW. Hip arthroscopy in athletes. Instr Course Lect 2003;52:701–9.
57. Byrd JW, Jones KS. Prospective analysis of hip arthroscopy with 2-year follow-up. Arthroscopy 2000;16(6):578–87.

Rehabilitation of the Spine Following Sports Injury

Eric Sampsell, PT, ATC

KEYWORDS

• Spine • Core • Athlete • Lumbar • Cervical

The spine is one of the most difficult areas of the body to both diagnose and treat, especially in the athlete. Injuries range from the insidious and mild to the catastrophic and severe. Although severe spinal injuries like fractures and dislocations are the most feared, most problems in the spine are due to loading and repetitive demands to the soft tissues, especially in impact sports. These are the injuries that will most commonly be seen by the physician, physical therapist, or athletic trainer. Although spinal pain is common in the general patient population, athletes may be affected by it at an equal or greater rate, limiting their function and decreasing sports performance. The complexity of movements, sport-specific biomechanics, and increased force generation may predispose the athlete to specific kinds of spinal injury, which is what makes treating the athlete with spinal pain much more challenging.

LUMBAR SPINE
Facet Joint Dysfunction

Facet joints (zygapophyseal joints) are commonly injured in athletes, especially after trauma. It has been reported that pain to the facet joint can be found in as many as 75% of people reporting low back pain (LBP).[1] The facet joint is covered by a highly innervated capsule that includes both proprioceptive and nociceptive nerve endings. Injury to this joint can include sprain, impingement of the capsule between the facet surfaces, and articular cartilage degeneration. A lack of mobility in the facets can lead to injury and is the most common reason for pain in the facet joint.[2]

Injury to the facet joint can arise from specific movements such as a side bending, rotation, or extension moment. Pure flexion tends to unload the facet joint and is usually not a major cause of injury by itself. Most athletic movements are multiplanar, and combinations of movements are more likely going to be the cause of facet injury. Axial rotation moments give the highest forces through the facet joint, more than doubling the forces produced by extension and almost tripling the forces of ipsilateral side bending.[3] In injuries to this joint, rotation seems to be the common element. A

WVUH-East City Hospital, 2000 Foundation Way, Martinsburg, WV 25401, USA
E-mail address: esampsell@cityhospital.org

Clin Sports Med 29 (2010) 127–156
doi:10.1016/j.csm.2009.09.011
0278-5919/09/$ – see front matter
sportsmed.theclinics.com

combination of hyperextension and rotation can be one of the most common mechanisms for facet joint pain (eg, tennis serve). The combined movements of flexion and rotation can also be a common mechanism (eg, rowing).

Subjective complaints from the athlete may include a feeling of "stiffness" or being "locked up"; typically, pain complaints are more common with rest, and tend to ease with movement and activity. The athlete will usually complain of nonradicular, localized pain adjacent to the spinous process, and range of motion may be significantly limited, especially in the early stages of injury. Two movement patterns may be apparent during the evaluation that reproduces pain. With extension, ipsilateral rotation, and side bending, the joint is compressed and pain may be elicited. With flexion, contralateral rotation, and side bending, the joint capsule is stretched, possibly causing pain (**Table 1**). Extension (eg, standing, walking, running) may aggravate symptoms as well, due to the higher loads placed on the joints. Pain is usually eased with flexion, especially in a seated position where there is essentially no load on the facet joints.[4] Tenderness and muscle spasm may be felt over the affected facet joint with palpation. From an imaging perspective, the best view to identify and assess the facet joints and pars interarticularis is the oblique radiograph, although an anteroposterior (AP) radiograph will show the facet joints as well.

Treatment

Early treatment goals for injury to the facet joint include pain relief and decreasing spasm; this can be done with gentle grade I and II mobilizations to the joint if it has been found to be hypomobile, soft tissue massage, modalities such as ultrasound and electrical stimulation, and gentle flexion based exercise. Avoiding extension in the early stages of healing is advised. Incorporating a light cardiovascular conditioning program during the early stages is important to promote movement and prevent deconditioning. Recumbent bicycle, aquatic therapy, and the use of an upper body ergometer may help to prevent deconditioning and avoid extension. This program can be progressed as the athlete's tolerance to movement and extension improves.

As muscle spasm and pain begin to subside, the aggressiveness of rehabilitation may increase, including traction in slight contralateral side bending and exercises that may have previously put undue stress on the facet joint. The addition of multiplanar movements with extension can be added to prepare the athlete for more sport-specific movements later in rehabilitation. Grade III and IV mobilizations can also be performed to regain mobility and restore lumbar range of motion (**Fig. 1**). Incorporating a structured core stability program with emphasis on transversus abdominis (TA) strengthening should be at the center of any low back program to address underlying

| Table 1 | |
| Normal facet function in the lumbar spine | |
Direction of Motion	Facet Function
Forward bending	Facets opens
Backward bending	Facets close
Side bending right	Right facet closes Left facet opens
Side bending left	Right facet opens Left facet closes

Data from Saunders D, Saunders Ryan R. Evaluation, treatment and prevention of musculoskeletal disorders. 4th edition. Chaska, MN: The Saunders Group; 2004. p. 274.

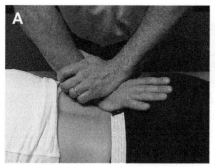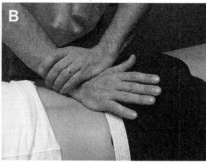

Fig. 1. (A) Lumbar left rotational mobilization with the use of the pisiform as contact point on transverse process. (B) PA mobilization of the spinous process in lumbar spine.

weaknesses that may have left the athlete vulnerable to injury. The facet joint capsule is highly innervated with proprioceptive nerve endings, so incorporating balance and sport-specific movements will be critical to returning the athlete to preinjury form.

Return to play

The amount of time lost will depend on severity of injury to the facet joint, and can range from 2 to 8 weeks. Before returning to play, the athlete should possess as close to possible pain-free active range of motion in all movements, especially with activities combining extension and rotation. Correcting poor mechanics and addressing overuse and overtraining will be important in preventing reoccurrence of the injury. Assessing for functional core strength and proprioception is critical, and the gradual progression of sport-specific activities should be assessed by the therapist or athletic trainer before releasing the athlete back to full competition.

Spondylolysis and Spondylolisthesis

Spondylolysis is a defect in the pars interarticularis, most commonly found at the L5-S1 segment in athletes. The mechanism for this injury is usually a result of repeated hyperextension moments, causing repeated stress through the pars interarticularis and a resultant stress fracture.[5] Although spondylolysis is usually unilateral in sports, the defect may become bilateral as the stress continues, causing the vertebrae to slip forward, resulting in spondylolisthesis. This forward slippage may narrow the spinal canal, possibly causing spinal cord impingement, most commonly at the level of L4-L5. Both injuries can be symptomatic, especially in the younger athletic population.[6] There are 5 classifications of these conditions (**Table 2**) as described by Wiltse, with isthmic being the most common in adolescent athletes.[7,8] Meyerding[9] proposed a classification system that is widely used to describe the amount of anterior translation a vertebral body has relative to the one below. The amount of slippage is measured as the percentage of the slipped vertebrae (**Table 3**).

The incidence of spondylolisthesis and spondylolysis in the general population is generally low, around 5%, but increases significantly in sports, especially in those requiring a lot of rotation and hyperextension. A study by Rossi and Dragoni[10] found the incidence rate to be as high as 40% in some sports (**Table 4**). Sports such as weightlifting, gymnastics, wrestling, diving, and the butterfly stroke in swimming have been associated with these injuries.

An athlete may present with unilateral LBP with local tenderness and a history of hamstring tightness. Hypermobility may be found at the segment suspected with

Table 2
Classification of spondylolysis and spondylolisthesis

Type	Description
I. Dysplastic	Congenital abnormalities
II. Isthmic	Stress fracture of the pars interarticularis
III. Degenerative	Degeneration of facet joints causing instability and possible slippage
III. Traumatic	Acute fracture in areas other than the pars interarticularis
IV. Pathologic	Bone disorder/disease causing breakdown of pars interarticularis

Data from Wiltse LL. Spondylolisthesis: classification and etiology. Symposium of the spine. Am Acad Orthop Surg 1969. p.143.

passive mobility testing. The one-legged extension test, whereby the subject stands on one leg and hyperextends the spine, can be performed to assess for possible pars interarticularis pathology (**Fig. 2**). If symptoms are reproduced, a diagnosis of spondylolysis may be indicated.

Diagnostic testing and imaging
Radiographs and computed tomography (CT) scans are limited due to the inability to detect the early phases of a pars defect that are not yet full fractures.[11,12] Oblique-view radiographs can be ordered to help detect a fracture at the collar area of the classic "Scotty Dog" deformity (**Fig. 3**A). The use of a single photon emission computed tomography bone scan (**Fig. 3**B) can help to identify acute stress reactions in the pars interarticularis, but may have difficulty in detecting older lyses.[13] Lateral radiographs may help to detect the presence of spondylolisthesis (**Fig. 3**C).

Treatment
After a diagnosis has been made, limiting the amount of extension the athlete performs is critical. Rest from all aggravating activities should be performed with consideration of an extension-limiting brace for 3 to 6 weeks. Rehabilitation can begin in the acute stages, with focus on pain relief through the use of modalities such as electrical stimulation, and education on postural control. Hip flexibility emphasizing hamstring and hip flexor stretching should be performed, with concentration on avoiding increased lordosis at the lumbar spine. Gentle mobilization of the segments above and below the affected joint may be beneficial for pain control and prevention of hypomobility at those segments.

As the athlete progresses into the subacute and chronic stages of healing, focus on core strengthening should be emphasized. Stimulation of the deep abdominal muscles in conjunction with the lumbar multifidus has been shown to help with pain

Table 3
Grades of spondylolisthesis

Grade 1	1%–25%
Grade 2	26%–50%
Grade 3	51%–75%
Grade 4	75%–100%
Grade 5	>100%

Data from Meyerding HW. Spondylolisthesis. J Bone Joint Surg 1931;13:39.

Table 4	
Incidence in spondylolisthesis and spondylolysis in athletes	
Sport	**Incidence Rate (%)**
Diving	40.4
Wrestling	25
Weightlifting	22.3
Modern pentathlon and triathlon in Track and Field	17.3
General population	5

Data from Rossi F, Dragoni S. The prevalence of spondylolysis and spondylolisthesis in symptomatic elite athletes: radiographic findings. Radiography 2001;7:37.

control in those with listhetic displacement.[14] As pain allows, progressing from static to more sport-specific exercise incorporating rotation and extension can be done, with emphasis on the TA and multifidus cocontraction.

Return to play
Return to sport may take up to 12 weeks or longer, depending on the severity of the injury. Restrictions will depend on signs and symptoms, and results of radiographs. If the athlete has an asymptomatic spondylolisthesis, he or she may return to sport with the use of a functional brace to limit hyperextension and rotation. If pain persists longer than 9 months, consideration for return to competition can be made by the

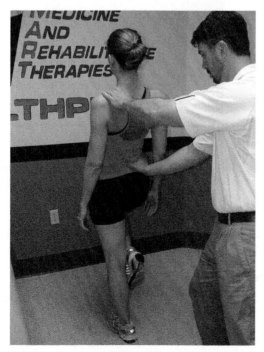

Fig. 2. The one-legged hyperextension test: The patient stands on one leg and hyperextends at the lumbar spine. Pain indicates possible spondylolysis.

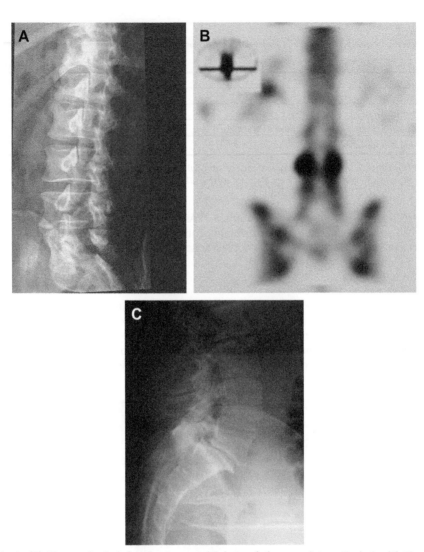

Fig. 3. (*A*) "Scotty dog" deformity in spondylolysis of the pars interarticularis. (*B*) Single photon emission computed tomography bone scan of a pars interarticularis fracture. (*C*) Radiograph of L5-S1 grade 1 to 2 spondylolisthesis.

physician. If pain continues to limit function and return to sport, surgery or modification in activity level may be required.[15]

Lumbar Disc Injuries

The intervertebral disc consists of the central nucleus pulposus that is encapsulated by a fibrous outer covering called the annulus. The disc can be injured through a single traumatic episode or over time through repetitive activity, with the most common site being at the L4-L5 or L5-S1 levels. The severity of injury can also vary from a small tear of the outer covering to a complete rupture of the annulus with portions of the nucleus pulposus lying outside the disc. The clean-and-jerk and squat during weight training are common exercises that may cause traumatic injury to an athlete's disc. Sports that commonly cause disc injuries include football, weightlifting, rowing, or any activity that may combine loading of the spine in combination with flexion or rotation.

Signs and symptoms are wide ranging and depend on the mechanism, location, and classification of the injury. Pain could present unilaterally or bilaterally, and with or without radiating pain into the buttock or lower extremity. If the nucleus has herniated out of the disc into the spinal canal, there will be both chemical and mechanical irritability, often causing unrelenting pain and a higher chance of neurologic symptoms such as parasthesia or myotomal weakness. Flexion, rotational, and loading positions will often aggravate the patient as well as any increase in intradiscal pressure such as coughing, sneezing, or a bowel movement. The presence of a lateral shift of the pelvis may be apparent, and is most commonly found away from the side of pain.[16]

If symptoms are present below the gluteal fold, a complete neurologic examination should be performed (**Table 5**). The physical examination may show motor weakness in the lower extremity, especially in ankle dorsiflexion (L4), great toe extension (L5), or plantarflexion of the ankle (S1). Dermatomal patterns of sensation loss should be noted, and the reflexes of the lower extremities checked for any changes and compared bilaterally (**Table 6**). It is important that clinicians be aware of the signs and symptoms of cauda equina syndrome when evaluating lumbar disc injuries. If the disc herniation is large enough, it may compress the nerve roots caudal to the level of spinal cord termination, causing parasthesia in the perianal region and loss of bowel or bladder control. This situation represents a medical emergency with immediate need to refer for possible surgical decompression.

Neural tension signs may be present, with a positive straight leg raise (SLR) or slump test that places tension on the L5-S3 nerve roots (**Fig. 4**). The SLR test is positive if symptoms are reproduced at an angle between 15° and 70°. A Crossed SLR test can be performed to the leg opposite to the radicular signs. If this test produces symptoms in the involved side, the result is very sensitive and specific for a herniated lumbar disc. When symptoms are on the anterior thigh, the femoral nerve stretch test can also be performed to test for femoral nerve irritability (**Fig. 5**).

Although the thoracic spine does not experience the same incidence of disc injury as the lumbar spine, the lower thoracic spine may be prone to degeneration in athletes who participate in sports that involve repetitive thoracic rotation, such as golf, baseball, and discus throwing. Pain is usually central, but may radiate along the ribcage following the thoracic nerve root with or without paresthesia. Extension and rotational movements may cause an aggravation of symptoms. Early mobilization and modalities may help to decrease pain, and focus on thoracic strengthening and stability should follow, with a gradual return to sport-specific activity.

Table 5
Components of the neurologic examination of lumbar spine

Sensory Testing	Myotome Testing	Reflex Testing
Inguinal area (L1)	Hip flexion (L1-L2)	Patellar tendon (L3-L4)
Proximal anterior thigh (L2)	Knee extension (L3-L4)	Achilles tendon (S1-S2)
Distal anterior thigh (L3)	Ankle dorsiflexion (L4-L5)	
Medial low leg (L4)	Great toe extension (L5)	
Lateral low leg (L5)	Ankle plantar flexion (S1-S2)	
Posterior calf (S1)		

Table 6
Clinical features of lumbar disc herniation

Findings	L3-4 Disc, L4 Nerve Root	L4-5 disc, L5 Nerve Root	L5-S1 Disc, S1 Nerve Root
Pain	Low back, hip, posterolateral thigh, across patella, anteromedial leg	SI region, hip, posterolateral thigh, anterolateral leg	SI region, hip, posterolateral thigh/leg
Numbness	Anteromedial thigh and knee	Lateral leg, first web space	Back of calf, lateral heel, foot, toe
Weakness	Knee extension	EHL (first ray extension)	Plantar flexion of ankle, first ray flexion
Atrophy	Quadriceps	Minimal anterior calf	Calf
Reflexes	L4 decreased	None of diagnostic significance	S1 diminished or absent

Data from Boden SD, Weisel SW, Laws ER, et al. The aging spine: essentials of pathophysiology, diagnosis, and treatment. 4th edition. Philadelphia: WB Saunders; 1997.

Diagnostic testing and imaging

Intervertebral disc space narrowing can be observed from AP and lateral radiographs, and sagittal and axial magnetic resonance imaging (MRI) can indicate a ruptured or herniated disc (**Fig. 6**). Some disc height loss may be normal in patients older than 35 to 40 years. The use of a myelogram can be used if spinal cord impingement is suspected.

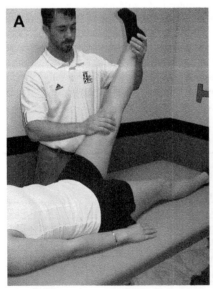 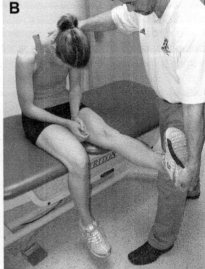

Fig. 4. (*A*) Straight leg raise test/crossed straight leg raise test. (*B*) Slump test.

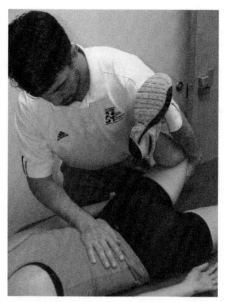

Fig. 5. Femoral nerve stretch test.

Treatment

The acute phase of a lumbar disc injury may last from 2 to 6 weeks, depending on the level of injury. The initial treatment should be focused on pain control and decreasing radicular symptoms out of the leg. The use of modalities such as transcutaneous electrical nerve stimulation (TENS), heat, and ultrasound may help initially to manage pain. Simple positioning in side-lying with the affected side up and cushioning under the down side may help to open the space and relieve symptoms (**Fig. 7**). Functional taping to limit flexion may be helpful and might also give proprioceptive feedback to the athlete to facilitate good posture (**Fig. 8**). The concept of "centralizing" pain should be used, assessing for positions and activities that help to alleviate radiating symptoms in the extremities. If radicular and neurologic symptoms appear as the primary complaint in the early stages of therapy, the use of traction may be useful to unload the disc.[17] Traction should initially be assessed manually, later progressing to the use of mechanical traction or floating traction in a pool if there is no increase in symptoms (**Fig. 9**). Early walking and aquatic therapy may help alleviate pain and allow the athlete to help prevent further deconditioning.

The use of McKenzie's program to help regain range of motion and decrease radicular symptoms may be appropriate, unless pain is worsened. There are 3 basic stages of the program: (1) correction of the shift or deformity, (2) prone lying with passive extension, and (3) generalized stretches incorporating some flexion and rotation. The program theorizes using extension to return the bulge back into the disc and to centralize the patient's symptoms.

As the athlete progresses to the subacute stages of injury (weeks 3–12), incorporation of further mobilization, stretching, and strengthening can be performed, emphasizing core stability. Particular emphasis should be placed on the lumbar spine and hip extensors. In the core program, initially neutral spine position should be emphasized, avoiding excessive flexion, rotation, and loaded positions. As the athlete improves, progression to more dynamic core stability exercises should be done,

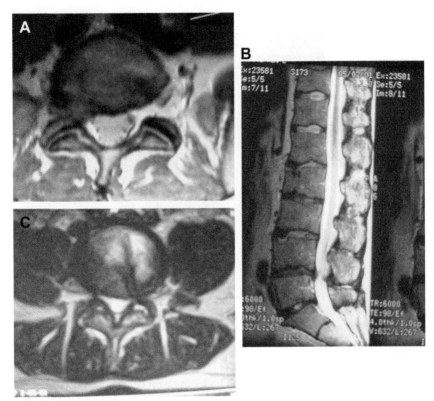

Fig. 6. (*A*) Magnetic resonance image (MRI) of a new L5-S1 left herniated disc. (*B*) MRI of L4-5 recurrent herniated disc, sagittal view. (*C*) Axial MRI of L4-5 left paracentral herniated disc.

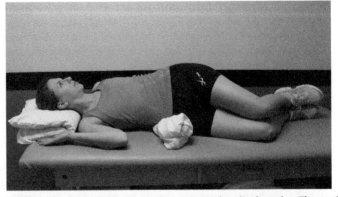

Fig. 7. Positioning for comfort with acute disc pain and radiculopathy. The patient lies in a side-lying position with the affected side up and a pillow placed under the hips. If tolerable, the patient can roll into slight rotation toward the side of pain to help open the foraminal space.

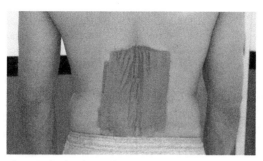

Fig. 8. Functional taping to the lumbar spine.

incorporating exercises that take the patient out of the neutral position. This activity will prepare athletes for the more functional activities and positions that they will need to tolerate when they return to play.

Return to play

Several studies have shown through serial MRIs that there is gradual resorption and disappearance of herniated discs without the use of surgical intervention. Up to 50% of patients with confirmed herniated nucleus pulposus will recover without surgery in 1 to 6 months.[15]

If surgery is required, single-level discectomies have shown that 90% of elite athletes will return to their sport.[18] For the athlete to return to play, they should have pain-free range of motion, full functional strength, and the ability to pass sport-specific drills and testing by the therapist or athletic trainer. The core stabilizers of the spine and hips should be evaluated thoroughly to ensure proper support to the spine. Possible modification to mechanics and emphasis on neutral spine should be given, especially in sports such as rowing that require a high degree of disc loading. It is advised that after any disc injury the athlete incorporates a core stability program in his or her regular routine, to try to minimize risk of further damage and degeneration that may inhibit sport or function in the future.

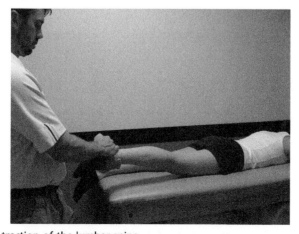

Fig. 9. Manual traction of the lumbar spine.

Lumbar Sprain and Strain

Sprains and strains to the spine are one of the more common injuries to the athlete who suffers from back pain. Due to the difficulty in differentiating between a sprain and a strain, they are usually grouped together when describing any injury to the soft tissue of the spine that includes ligaments, muscle, tendon, or the musculotendinous junction. Signs and symptoms may include paraspinal muscle spasm, or tenderness without radiculopathy and localized bruising. If pain is referred to the hips or buttocks, thoracodorsal fascial injury may be present due to its connection to the tensor fascia lata. Painful and limited range of motion will most likely be present, particularly with rotation and flexion. Pain will ease with rest and be aggravated with activity. When severe bruising is present with a traumatic mechanism of injury, fracture or renal injury should be suspected, particularly with the presence of hematuria. With sprains and strains, radiographs will be negative. MRI is not normally needed, but should be considered if neurologic signs are present or symptoms do not improve.

Treatment

Depending on the level of irritability, a period of inactivity or bed rest may be necessary. Mild stretching, cryotherapy, and soft tissue massage can be used as the first line of treatment. The use of modalities such as ultrasound and TENS can be useful in decreasing spasm and pain. Although not studied in the athletic population, active treatment including exercise has been shown to be ineffective in the general population with acute LBP.[19] The use of low-level grade I and II joint mobilizations may help in decreasing pain and spasm. Performing low-level movements in a pool may allow the athlete to maintain some level of conditioning during the injury process, as well as decreasing muscle spasm and pain. If thoracolumbar fascial injury is suspected or muscle spasm is present, soft tissue massage and myofascial release techniques such as fascial rolling may help to increase mobility and minimize symptoms **(Fig. 10)**. The use of aspirin, nonsteroidal anti-inflammatory drugs (NSAIDS), and acetaminophen can be useful, with muscle relaxers and opioids being seldom used with sprains and strains.

Assessment of hip and spinal joint mobility will be important due to increased likelihood of injury later if restriction is present. Assessment of neural tension will be needed and may be a source of pain. Performing light neural glides in the early stages of treatment may help, later performing more aggressive neural glides in the subacute

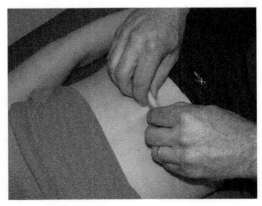

Fig. 10. Fascial rolling to increase mobility of the lumbar spine.

and chronic stages of injury. Performing grade III and IV joint mobilizations to hypomobile segments may help in treating the current injury and may help to prevent future injuries. As soon as the patient is able to tolerate exercise, performing a core stabilization program with emphasis on hip, lumbar, and abdominal musculature is critical. Not only is there going to be loss of strength and proprioception to this area, there may be a need to treat underlying weakness that may have contributed to the injury. As pain allows, exercise will progress to more functional and sport-specific activity.

Return to play

A typical sprain/strain may take from a few days to several weeks to heal properly and allow for return to sports. The athlete should present with full active and pain-free range of motion of lumbar spine as well as be able to perform all sport-specific tasks pain-free. Proper core strength should be present and all biomechanical problems should be corrected before returning to competition.

CERVICAL SPINE
Cervical Fracture and Dislocations

In the athletic population, most cervical spine injuries are not serious and are generally soft tissue in nature. Fractures of the cervical spine are not common, but are considered medical emergencies that should be referred immediately to a specialist. Fractures and dislocations of the cervical spine are most common in football and are usually caused by 1 of 3 different mechanisms, hyperflexion, hyperextension, and axial compression (eg, spearing), with axial compression being cited as the force most responsible for serious cervical spine injury in football.[20] Spearing has been associated with Jefferson fractures, a bilateral fracture of the ring of C1 (**Fig. 11**). Poor tackling mechanics are a cause for this injury, and education in proper form should be a priority for all medical professionals and coaches to their team at the start of the season. Serious injury should be assumed in any cervical spine injury that is traumatic in nature and includes any of the mechanisms described here. They should also be considered serious if they present with any signs of neurologic impairment or concussion (**Table 7**).

The location of the fracture will determine the seriousness and the treatment of the injury. Upper cervical spine fractures at C1-C2 should be considered separately from those in the lower cervical spine due to the unique anatomy at these levels. Spinous and transverse process fractures, though painful and significantly limiting the range

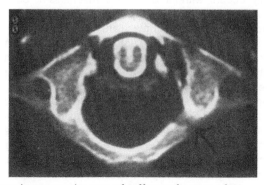

Fig. 11. Axial computed tomography scan of Jefferson fracture of C1.

Table 7
Components of the neurologic examination of cervical spine

Sensory Testing	Myotome Testing	Reflex Testing
Lateral arm (C5)	Deltoid (C5)	Biceps (C5)
Thumb (C6)	Wrist Ext (C6)	Brachioradialis (C6)
Middle finger (C7)	Tricep (C7)	Triceps (C7)
Fifth finger (C8)	Finger flexion (C8)	
Medial forearm (T1)	Interossei (T1)	

of motion, most likely will not cause paralysis or spinal cord injury compared with vertebral body fractures or dislocations.

Unless radiographs have cleared the athlete of fracture or dislocation after traumatic injury, the evaluation process should be cautious and nonaggressive. Further movement of an unstable vertebral segment or bone fragments by range of motion testing and palpation may cause further damage to the spinal cord. If fracture or dislocation is suspected, immediate immobilization and referral to the emergency facility should be performed. The open-mouth odontoid radiograph historically has been the most common view used to diagnose fractures at C1. CT and MRI have been used more recently for more definitive diagnosis for C1, with the MRI helping to determine tearing of the transverse ligament.

Treatment
Whether the fracture is stable or unstable will determine the treatment. If stable, most fractures with be treated with a rigid collar for 8 to 12 weeks. If unstable, a fracture in the cervical spine may require fusion (C2 or lower) or halo immobilization (C1). The rehabilitation will be determined by the level of dysfunction following injury, and will focus on activities of daily life and return to a functional standard of living.

Return to play
Due to the catastrophic nature of this injury, it is most likely that the athlete will not return to contact sports. Depending on the level of neurologic impairment and spinal cord trauma, the athlete may return to such recreational activities such as golfing, walking, or cycling, with physician approval.

Acute Cervical Painful Entrapment

A painful entrapment refers to unilateral pain and stiffness in a cervical facet joint. The entrapment usually occurs without a specific mechanism, but may present the morning after a bout of heavy upper body activity or prolonged awkward positioning of the head. Overloading the shoulder musculature that attaches to the cervical spine and facet joints is usually the cause of the entrapment. The athlete may report waking in the morning with a stiff neck or even feeling a "pop" after a sudden movement of the head. Pain and stiffness worsens over the next few hours accompanied by loss of range of motion, especially toward the painful side.

Upon evaluation, range of motion will be limited in ipsilateral rotation and side bending. Flexion may aggravate symptoms if the facet entrapment is in the lower cervical spine, with extension being limited and painful in upper cervical spine facet entrapments. Pain beyond the shoulder is not common, indicating a more accurate diagnosis of a soft tissue restriction within the facet joint capsule. Trigger points and muscle spasm throughout the upper trapezius, levator scapula, rhomboids, and suprascapular region will be common and a result of the entrapment.

Assessment of posture and strength testing of the deep anterior neck flexors and posterior neck musculature should be performed, which may point to the underlying cause of the injury. Weak anterior neck flexors can be assessed by asking the athlete to lay supine and raise the head from the table. If the athlete leads his or her head forward with the chin, this may indicate weakness in the deep anterior neck flexors (**Fig. 12**). Weaknesses in these deep stabilizing muscles may cause minor instability, resulting in shortening of the levator scapula and upper trapezius muscles. This shortening could cause spasm or chronic trigger points. Chronically poor posture presenting with forward head and rounded shoulders with increased thoracic kyphosis may lead an athlete to be more prone to a painful entrapment.

If the underlying weaknesses and postural syndrome are not addressed, the athlete may become prone to more frequent bouts of a painful entrapment. The facet joint capsule may become thickened and scarred, possibly causing longer bouts of limitations and dysfunction, leading to possible permanent restriction in range of motion. Unless the athlete presents with traumatic mechanism and signs of neurologic involvement, a true painful entrapment usually does not require the use of any imaging. If pain persists and therapy has not been successful, radiographs should be performed especially if a hard end feel is noted.[21]

Treatment

The pain may initially be severe enough that the use of modalities such as continuous ultrasound, moist heat, and electrical stimulation may be the only treatment options. Soft tissue massage can also be used to help decrease muscle spasm and trigger points. A physician may prescribe analgesics, NSAIDS, or muscle relaxants in the initial stages of the entrapment. After the first 24 to 48 hours of the injury, the acute inflammatory process should begin to resolve, and the initiation of passive cervical range of motion and stretching can be performed by either the therapist or athlete. At this point, stiffness may be the prominent symptom rather than resting pain, although pain will be present with active movement. The use of self- or therapist-directed isometric rotation to the painful side in multiple ranges may help to "free" the entrapment (**Fig. 13**).

It is key to focus on restoring mobility to the affected facet joint. If the focus of therapy is on treating the spasm and trigger points, pain may continue as these are the result of the underlying restriction and not usually the primary injury. Cervical mobilization can be performed, immediately focusing on the segments above and below the restriction, for pain relief and to prevent further limitations. Grade I and II mobilizations can be done at the painful segment for pain relief, progressing to grade III and IV mobilizations to increase mobility as pain allows. Mobilizations can be performed at

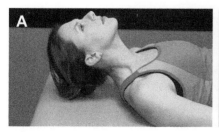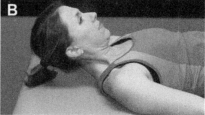

Fig. 12. Test for weakness of deep cervical flexors. The athlete is asked to raise her head from the table. (*A*) A positive test is found when the athlete leads with the chin, indicating weakness in deep anterior neck flexors. (*B*) Normal test.

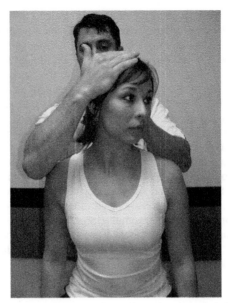

Fig. 13. Cervical contract-relax technique. The patient shown lacks left cervical rotation. The patient is placed in position toward the restricted movement and is asked to rotate her head to the right.

the segment(s) found to be restricted in a prone or seated position, depending on the comfort of the athlete. The use of facet downgliding in an oblique plane or posterior to anterior mobilizations should be performed on the side of restriction.

Long-term correction of posture and postural weakness should be performed through therapeutic exercises. Strengthening the often weak deep anterior neck flexors should be performed initially with light isometrics (**Fig. 14**). Progression to higher-level range of motion and strengthening exercises should be added as strength goals are met and pain allows.

Return to play
The athlete may return to sport-specific activity as pain allows and as functional range of motion is regained. Continued education in proper posture and exercises designed

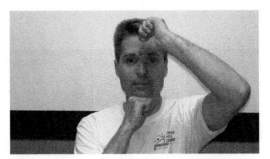

Fig. 14. Strengthening of the deep anterior neck flexors. The patient is asked to place 1 to 2 finger tips onto the forehead while in good cervical posture. The patient is told to press *lightly* onto the forehead and perform an isometric contraction. The motion should mimic upper cervical spine flexion or nodding.

to provide stability to the cervical spine should continue even as the athlete returns to sport, to help prevent reoccurrence of the injury.

Headaches

It has been reported that up to a third of university athletes have experienced exercise-related headaches at some point in their career.[22] Williams and Nukada developed 4 categories of sport headaches; effort migraine, trauma-triggered migraine, effort-exertion headache, and posttraumatic headache. The 2 most common were effort-exertion headache (60%) and posttraumatic headache (22%). Women were found to more commonly suffer from effort-related headaches following activities like jogging, whereas men in contact sports suffered from more trauma-induced headache, such as in a collision in football or hockey.

In nontraumatic headaches, continuous extension of the upper cervical spine may cause spasm and pressure to the suboccipital nerve. Cyclists and athletes who have continuously poor postural habits may be prone to these headaches. Patients may present with very tight and tender suboccipital muscles, preexisting cervical facet restrictions, and weakness in the deep anterior neck flexors. Facet joints may be very tender unilaterally or bilaterally, and pain may be severe enough to inhibit function. If headache is chronic or severe, initial bloodwork can be performed to help rule out metabolic causes of headaches. CT scan, MRI/magnetic resonance angiography, or angiogram studies are indicated if the athlete describes the headache to be the first or worse headache of his or her life, if the headache persists or progresses, or if there is an abnormal neurologic examination.[23]

Treatment

The use of moist heat to the posterior cervical spine can begin treatment and relax the athlete. Soft tissue mobilization to the suboccipital region can be performed with gentle grade I and II facet glides in an anterior to posterior direction. If tolerable, the use of grade III or IV anterior mobilizations to the spinous process of C2 can be performed in a supine or prone position (**Fig. 15**). Lateral glides of the transverse process can be performed at C2 and may help decrease symptoms (**Fig. 16**). Performing a suboccipital release may be of benefit if the athlete presents with excessive hyperextension of the upper cervical spine, and has suboccipital tenderness and tightness. Mobilization to restricted cervical facets can be done, and stretching of the suboccipitals muscle group may help prevent pressure to the suboccipital nerve. Treating

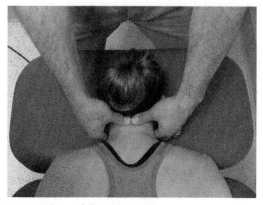

Fig. 15. Cervical posteroanterior mobilization to C2.

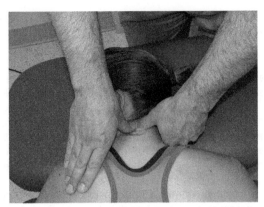

Fig. 16. Lateral glide onto transverse process of upper cervical spine for headache on left side of the head.

poor postural habits in the athlete and assessing the athlete's ergonomics (eg, bike position, handlebars) may help in preventing further recurrent headaches.

Return to play

If the headache is a result of trauma there may have been a concussion, and assessment by a specialist should be performed before returning to sport. If a concussion is suspected, all signs and symptoms should be resolved, and clearance by the attending physician should be given before returning to sport. If the headache is of a nontraumatic nature, the athlete may participate as long as he or she presents with normal neurologic assessment and symptoms do not worsen.

REHABILITATION APPROACHES FOR SPINE REHABILITATION
Williams Flexion

The flexion-biased program was developed in 1937 by Dr Paul Williams to not only reduce pain, but to also provide trunk stability by strengthening the abdominals, gluteals, and hamstrings. Passive stretching of the hip flexors and low back muscles were also at the center of his program, with the ultimate goal of providing a balance between the flexors and extensors that provide postural stability.

These exercises currently are commonly used for patients who present with pain originating from the posterior elements of the spine, such as a with facet joint syndrome (**Fig. 17**). During the evaluation process, the patients who would benefit from this program are those who show symptomatic relief or a centralization of their pain with repetitive flexion movements. Although these exercises may be beneficial in some cases, patients who present with acute disc herniation should avoid flexion due to the increase in intradiscal pressure that comes with flexion of the lumbar spine. There has been little consensus about specific protocol for these exercises, but individualized progression is the goal.

Research and Flexion-Based Exercise

The concern with flexion-based exercise is the increase in intradiscal pressure, which could aggravate those patients with herniated or bulging discs. In 1981 Nachemson[24] determined that the full sit-up exercise in Williams' program increased intradiscal pressure 210% compared with a standing position, with 3 of the 6 exercises becoming contraindicated for those with acute herniated discs. It has been found that early

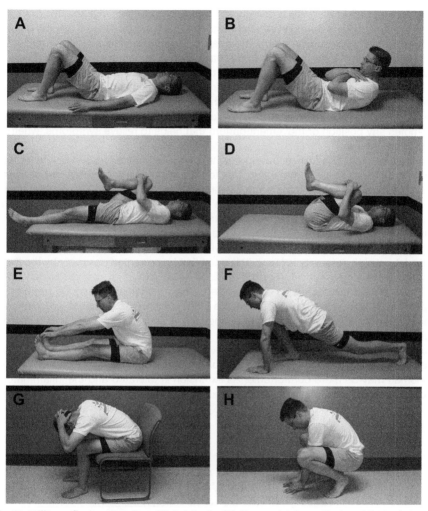

Fig. 17. Williams flexion exercises. (*A*) Pelvic tilt. (*B*) Sit up with knee flexion. (*C*) Single knee to chest. (*D*) Double knee to chest. (*E*) Hamstring and erector spinae stretch. (*F*) Hip flexor stretch. (*G*) Seated flexion. (*H*) Squat for quadriceps strengthening.

morning flexion exercises may increase symptoms of nonspecific and chronic LBP in patients compared with a control group who performed "sham" exercises that have been shown to be ineffective in treating LBP. Due to an increase in disc fluid in the morning, increased lumbar flexion, especially standing toe touches, may aggravate symptoms and were not advised for those experiencing chronic LBP.[25] Repeated flexion-based exercises may help to centralize pain in those who are experiencing pain from facet joint syndrome by reducing facet joint compression. Flexion-based exercise may help to alleviate spasm in lumbar musculature and may stretch ligamentous and myofascial structures.[15]

Extension Theory

Robin McKenzie noted that some patients responded well to positions of extension, going against the strong theory and practice of Williams' flexion exercises at the time. He developed diagnostic categories that placed patients in a specific program based on the findings during evaluation, with the likelihood that they would be placed into an extension-biased program. The goals of these exercises are to centralize the pain of the patient from the limbs to the back. The phenomenon of centralization of pain with extension may be explained by the displacement of the intradiscal mass, relieving stress of structures that are causing referred pain in the limbs.[26] Due to the success that the McKenzie program has achieved in treating acute LBP with extension exercises, it has been labeled an "extension program." In fact, McKenzie's method promotes any position or movement pattern that helps to relieve symptoms, whether flexion or extension.

McKenzie classifies LBP according to how pain responds to specific movement patterns and positions of the spine. This identification of a movement or positional pattern that relieves symptoms is the defining characteristic of the McKenzie system. A patient may be classified as having a postural syndrome, a derangement, or a dysfunction, each having a particular treatment regimen that includes postural education and correction. Recognizing the correct pattern or mechanical diagnosis is critical in determining which exercises will be most effective.

If a lateral shift deformity is found, this must first be corrected passively by the therapist or by the athlete actively (**Fig. 18**). As soon as the pattern of exercise is found that will alleviate symptoms and centralize them, the movement should be performed repetitively. The first few repetitions may be more irritating to the patient, so emphasis on slow and passive movements to end range are important. When prone extension is being used, the therapist should have the patient focus on relaxation of the gluteal muscles to help ensure a more passive movement. Too much range of motion initially may increase symptoms, so starting in a prone lying position with pillows under the abdomen may be more comfortable. As extension is tolerated and the inflammatory process improves, increasing extension exercises can be performed, with focus on

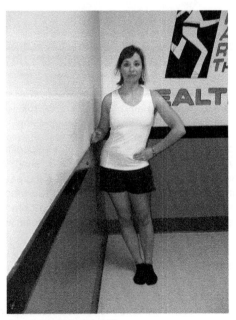

Fig. 18. Self correction for a right lateral shift.

centralizing pain (**Fig. 19**). Centralizing pain occurs most frequently with repeated extension movements and occasionally with lateral movements. Centralization only rarely occurs with flexion.

Research and Extension Theory

It has been reported that 87% of patients with radiating pain were able to centralize their pain during the first 48 hours.[26] McKenzie states that 98% of patients with symptoms of less than 4 weeks duration who experienced centralization of their pain on the first day of treatment had excellent to good results. This number decreases to 77% for those patients with subacute symptoms between 4 and 12 weeks. Most patients will centralize their pain in the first 2 days or sooner of treatment, with those experiencing centralization having a better outcome.

Adams and colleagues[27] found that the use of extension can reduce the stress of the posterior annulus of the disc, a common source of discogenic pain. Pain relief may be limited by the height of the disc and the shape of the neural arch. Those patients with significant degeneration of their discs with decreased disc height may not have as much relief as those with no history of change in disc height. It is also important that there are no reproducible data suggesting that exercise can move the nucleus pulposus.[28] Ingber[28] states that another explanation of symptom relief

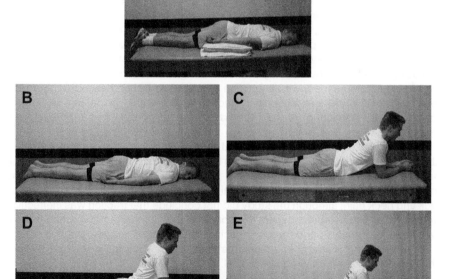

Fig. 19. Progression of lumbar extension positions. (*A*) Prone with support under abdomen. (*B*) Prone with no support. (*C*) Prone on elbows. (*D*) Prone on hands. (*E*) Prone extension performed with belt.

with extension-based exercises may be associated with elongation of the iliopsoas muscles and hip flexors.

If the goal of the therapist is to perform a truly passive treatment for the athlete, lying prone without movement will elicit the least amount of activity in the erectors. Feibert found that even passive movements in a prone position into extension have been found to activate lumbar back extensors.[29]

In 1998 Cherkin and colleagues[30] concluded that neither chiropractic manipulation nor McKenzie back exercises provided a significant functional benefit compared with a placebo group that received an educational booklet on LBP. The McKenzie exercises were found to have a slightly greater level of pain relief than the placebo. It is critical to underscore that these exercises did not include the inclusion of a core stability program. Two studies have shown that low back stiffness may only be a symptom of LBP and not the direct cause of it.[31–33] Johannsen et al[31] concluded that increased spinal mobility does not necessarily lead to LBP improvement, and that mobilizing exercises alone should not be recommended to those patients with LBP.

Traction

Traction may help to alleviate pain by providing muscle relaxation, stimulating mechanoreceptors, and inhibiting reflexive muscle guarding.[31] Traction can be used to treat herniated or degenerative discs, as well as hypomobile joints. Traction can be applied intermittently or continuously, and can be applied manually or mechanically. In the treatment of mechanical neck pain, a systematic review in 2006 on mechanical traction recommended the clinical use of intermittent traction over continuous traction.[34] The use of intermittent traction historically has been used more with general pain, and continuous traction more with nerve root impingement and radicular symptoms.

To determine whether traction is an appropriate course of treatment, the clinician can apply manual traction to the neck while the patient is in a seated or supine position. In the lumbar spine, one of the lower extremities can be gently pulled while the patient is in a supine or prone position. If symptoms are not aggravated, the use of mechanical traction may be beneficial as the acuteness of the injury subsides, increasing the force of pull as they improve. Using a neutral position at the affected segment is recommended, with a position of increased flexion needed to get to the lower segments of the cervical spine. Traction to the lumbar spine can be done in a supine 90-90 position, or prone if the patient has responded well to an extension program.

Although widely used in the clinic to treat a variety of spinal injuries, there has been little evidence to support the use of traction in the literature. There is also little research that discusses the use of traction on the athletic population. Van der Heijden and colleagues[35] found that there was no real conclusion on the effects of traction on back and neck pain, although the study did not conclude that traction was ineffective. Although studies have been generally inconclusive, it is important to note that there have been few studies performed on specifically diagnosed injuries. Traction can be a useful adjunct to therapy in specific patients who are clinically relevant and for whom decompression would be beneficial.

Manual Therapy and the Spine

Manual therapy techniques are specific passive movements that are placed onto a hypomobile joint to restore motion, or in a joint that is moving normally to decrease pain. Soft tissue massage, passive stretching, and the use of muscle energy techniques are also used to increase mobility of soft tissue structures, but may not be as successful in increasing joint mobility. Joint mobilizations can be used and are effective throughout various ranges of motion, allowing the patient to be placed in a more comfortable position. These movements are usually graded from I to V, with grade V being labeled a high-velocity thrust that should only be performed by specially trained therapists (**Table 8**). Grades I and II are used in more acute conditions and for pain relief, with grades III and IV generally used in more chronic conditions and for increasing joint mobility.

The clinical effectiveness of manual therapy techniques continues to be controversial, with many differing conclusions. The literature does seem to justify the use of manual therapy for certain spinal problems, with the key being the use of sound clinical judgment. Serious side effects have been reported in the literature, including local discomfort, headache, dizziness, and even vertebral artery dissection resulting from high-velocity manipulation.[36] One study compared the use of high-velocity thrust maneuvers to mobilizations in the cervical spine, and concluded that mobilization was as effective in reducing neck pain and disability.[36] Due to the increased risk of high-velocity thrust manipulation, the use of joint mobilizations seems to be a safer and equally effective treatment.

Neural Tension and Back Pain

The concepts of manual therapy, exercise therapy, and joint mobilization have been around and in use for many years, with a majority of the research focusing on these forms of treatment. The concept of neurodynamics or neural tension has not stood alone as a form of treatment. This concept has been integrated into other treatment programs and assessment tools as an adjunct to "traditional therapy". Primary neural tension injuries are rare, but symptoms of increased mechanical traction to the nerve can be a result of a previous severe back injury, and may be a cause of chronic back or leg pain.[37]

The slump test and SLR test can be performed to determine if neural tension is a factor in the athlete's pain. The sciatic nerve may be tractioned further by placing the athlete in a full SLR position, adding hip adduction and ankle dorsiflexion and inversion (**Fig. 20**). Some athletes may have mild, recurrent episodes of LBP due to tight posterior neurologic structures that will only be found when the sciatic nerve is fully stretched. These athletes may complain of LBP during the end of their stride in their lead leg during a full sprint. If neural tension is found, incorporating gentle mobilization initially of the nervous system may be beneficial. Initial exercises may include simple short-arc quadriceps exercises for the knee or dorsiflexion range of motion at the ankle. As the acuteness of the pain improves, combining an element of spinal

Table 8	
Joint mobilization grades	
Grade I	Slow, small-amplitude movements performed at the beginning of the range
Grade II	Slow, large-amplitude movements performed through the range, but not reaching end range
Grade III	Slow, large-amplitude movements performed at limits of range
Grade IV	Slow, small-amplitude movements performed at the limit of the range and into resistance
Grade V	Fast, small-amplitude, high-velocity movement performed beyond the pathologic limit of the range

Data from Maitland G. Vertebral manipulation. 5th edition. Boston: Butterworths; 1986.

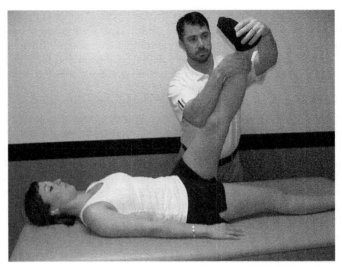

Fig. 20. Progressive stretch of the sciatic nerve performed with addition of hip adduction and ankle dorsiflexion, and inversion to the SLR position.

flexion to stretch the lumbosacral nerves or hip extension and knee flexion to glide the femoral or upper lumbar spinal nerves can be done.

These stretches can be done after a proper warm-up, with specific instruction to the athlete on avoiding pain while performing neural glides early in the healing process. If a painful stretch is pushed through, exacerbation of the pain may occur. The athlete should be instructed to stretch to the point of tension or discomfort, not through the pain. As the injury becomes chronic, the stretches can become more aggressive, stretching through the tension, as long as symptoms are not aggravated.

Lumbar Stabilization or Core Stability

After a low back injury, research has shown that the stabilizing musculature of the lumbar spine can show decreases in strength, coordination, size, and density, as well as show decreased activation.[38] The literature supports that improving core stability after an injury can lead to improvements in LBP. The goal of any core stability program is to strengthen the musculature that stabilizes the trunk, incorporating cocontraction of the abdominals. The core will then act as a corset, supporting and stabilizing the spine. The core stabilizers of the spine include not only the multifidi, erector spinae, and abdominals but also the lower extremity musculature of the hip. The functions of these core muscles are to oppose movements of the arms and legs, stabilize the spine, and decrease lumbar shearing. The TA has been shown to act to stabilize the spine even before limb motion occurs.[39,40]

Assessing athletes' ability to stabilize their core in a non-weight bearing position can be done initially during the early stages of the rehabilitation process. This assessment can be done by evaluating lumbopelvic motion in a supine or prone position, looking for excessive movement or decreased mobility with a pelvic tilt. Assessing the athlete's ability to find and maintain a neutral spine position between full anterior and posterior tilt of the pelvis can also help in assessing core strength (**Fig. 21**).

Although it is widely accepted that training the core will impact the effects of back pain, the literature is unclear as to which exercises are best to rehabilitate the athlete

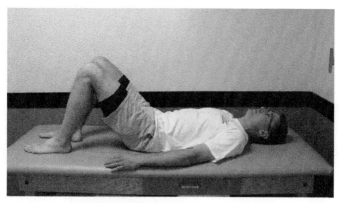

Fig. 21. Assessing ability to achieve neutral position.

back to the preinjury level of function. Several studies discuss electromyography (EMG) results of the core stabilizers during specific exercise, but most of the EMG studies have limitations because they are done with surface electrodes, making it difficult to measure the true amplitude of the response to activation. The athlete initially should begin with more unloaded exercises to isolate the TA and the multifidi while attempting to maintain the neutral position (**Figs. 22** and **23**). Athletes have a tendency to

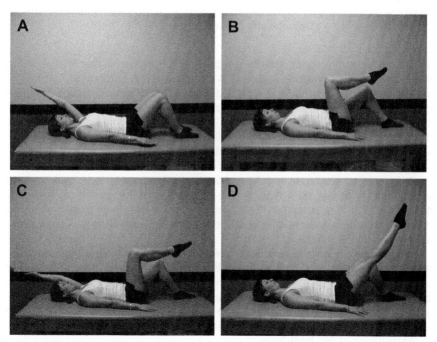

Fig. 22. Stabilization exercises in a supine unloaded position while maintaining neutral spine position and transversus abdominis (TA) contraction. (*A*) Alternating upper extremity movement. (*B*) Alternating lower extremity movement. (*C*) Opposite alternating upper and lower extremity movement. (*D*) Straight leg raise maintaining neutral spine position with TA contraction.

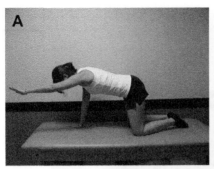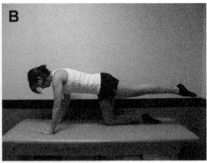

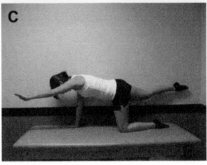

Fig. 23. Stabilization exercises performed in quadruped position. All exercises focus on neutral spine position and maintaining contraction of TA. (*A*) Alternating arm raises. (*B*) Alternating leg raises. (*C*) Opposite arm and leg raises.

overuse their external abdominal obliques, and often perform higher level exercises without the ability to stabilize properly in neutral with TA contraction. This action can be carried out isometrically in supine, quadruped, and prone positions, progressing to the addition of upper and lower extremity movement, and eventually to more loading and functional positions (**Fig. 24**). Throughout every exercise, it is critical to emphasize neutral spine as well as the ability to maintain a normal breathing pattern, avoiding increasing intradiscal pressure with the Valsalva maneuver.

As soon as the athlete can tolerate it, he or she should then be assessed more functionally in a closed-chain position. A functional and effective way to test the core is by performing a single-leg squat (**Fig. 25**). The athlete is asked to balance on one leg and squat down as low as possible. The clinician should look for any breakdown of the core during this movement, such as trunk side bending, loss of balance, or excessive flexion/extension of the spine.

Watkins[41] developed a coordinated core program for the injured athlete that is divided into 5 levels of 8 categories. The program allows the patient to go from a controlled neutral spine position to advanced strength exercises that require further balance and coordination. Some categories can potentially advance faster than others based on pain level, strength, and ability to maintain TA contraction and stability. The program also incorporates a diversified aerobic conditioning subprogram, critical to the rehabilitation of any back injury.

There is currently no standard of testing the core to ensure safe criteria for return to play after injury to the spine, although Watkins has established 5 criteria for returning to sport. Performing the single-leg squat test, and monitoring progress in time and breakdown of stability in multiple plank positions may help to give an idea of core

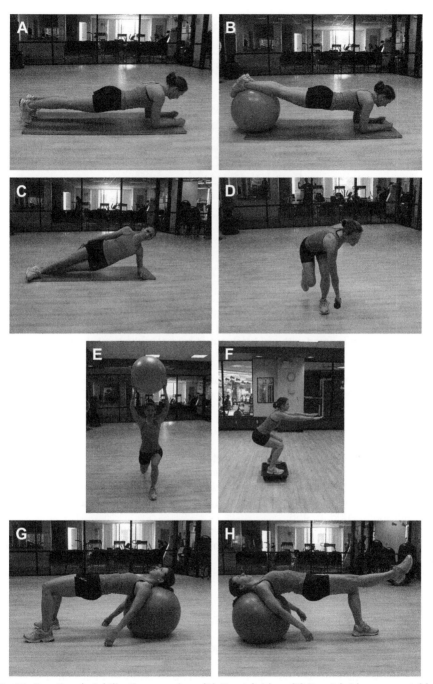

Fig. 24. Functional stabilization exercises. (*A*) Front bridge. (*B*) Front bridge on unstable surface. (*C*) Side bridge. (*D*) One-legged rotational squat. (*E*) Lunge with overhead movement. (*F*) Squat on rocker board. (*G*) Bridge on unstable surface. (*H*) Bridge on unstable surface with alternating leg lift.

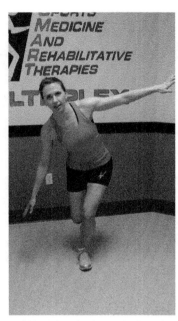

Fig. 25. Single-leg squat test. Athlete is asked to stand in single-leg position and perform a squat. Weakness is noted with any break out of neutral at the trunk, hips, or knees.

strength in the athlete. Having the athlete perform pain-free sport-specific drills while maintaining proper mechanics is critical to minimizing the chance of reinjury.

REFERENCES

1. Manchikanti L, Pampati V, Fellow B, et al. The inability of the clinical picture to characterize pain from facet joints. Pain Physician 2003;3:158–66.
2. Houglum P, Taylor B. Lumbar spine injuries. In: Starkey C, Johnson G, editors. Athletic training and sports medicine. Sudbary (MA): Jones and Bartlett Publishers; 2006. p. 458.
3. Schmidt H, Heuer F, Claes L, et al. The relation between the instantaneous center of rotation and facet joint forces—a finite element analysis. Clin Biomech 2008; 23(3):270–9.
4. Adams MA, Hutton WC. The mechanical function of the lumbar apophyseal joints. Spine 1983;8:327–9.
5. Letts M, Smallman T, Afanasiev R, et al. Fracture of the pars interarticularis in adolescent athletes: a clinical biomechanical analysis. J Pediatr Orthop 1986;6: 40–6.
6. Standaert C. The diagnosis and management of lumbar spondylolysis. Oper Tech Sports Med 2005;13(2):101–7.
7. Gross M, Mandelbaum B. Spondylolysis and spondylolisthesis. In: Reider B, editor. Sports medicine: the school age athlete. 2nd edition. Philadelphia: WB Saunders; 1991.
8. Wiltse LL. Spondylolisthesis: classification and etiology. Symposium of the spine. J Am Acad Orthop Surg 1969. p. 143.
9. Meyerding HW. Spondylolisthesis. J Bone Joint Surg Am 1931;13:39–48.

10. Rossi F, Dragoni S. The prevalence of spondylolysis and spondylolisthesis in symptomatic elite athletes: radiographic findings. Radiography 2001;7:37.
11. Amato M, Totty WG, Gilula LA. Spondylolysis of the lumbar spine: demonstration of defects and laminal fragmentation. Radiology 1984;153(3):627–9.
12. Hession PR, Butt WP. Imaging of spondylolysis and spondylolisthesis. Eur Radiol 1996;6(3):284–90.
13. Saraste H, Nilsson B, Brostrom LA, et al. Relationship between radiological and clinical variables in spondylolysis. Int Orthop 1984;8(3):163–74.
14. O'Sullivan PB, Physty GD, Twomey LT, et al. Evaluation of specific stabilizing exercise in the treatment of chronic low back pain with radiologic diagnosis of spondylolysis or spondylolisthesis. Spine 1997;22:2959–67.
15. Brotzman B. Low back injuries. In: Brotzman B, Wilk K, editors. Clinical ortho-pedic rehabilitation. Philadelphia: Mosby; 2003. p. 557–8.
16. McKenzie RA. The lumbar spine: mechanical diagnosis and therapy. Waikanae, Wellington, New Zealand: Spinal Publications New Zealand Limited; 1981.
17. Maitland G, Hengeveld E, Banks K, et al. Vertebral manipulation. 6th edition. Oxford: Butterworth Heinemann; 2001.
18. Wang J, Shapiro M, Hatch J. The outcome of lumbar discectomy in elite athletes. Spine 1999;24(6):570–3.
19. Faas A, Battie MC, Malmivaara A. Exercises: which ones are worth trying, for which patients, and when? Spine 1996;21:2874–9.
20. Torg JS, Vesgo JJ, O'Neill MJ, et al. The epidemiological, pathologic, biomechan-ical and cinematographic analysis of football induced cervical spine trauma. Am J Sports Med 1990;18:50–7.
21. Wajswelner H. Spine. In: Kolt G, Snyder-Mackler L, editors. Physical therapies in sport and exercise. St Louis (MO): Elsevier Publishing; 2003. p. 240.
22. Williams SJ, Nukada H. Sport and exercise headache: part 2. Diagnosis and classification. Br J Sports Med 1994;28:96–100.
23. Silberstein SD, Lipton RB. Overview of diagnosis and treatment of migraine. Neurology 1994;44(10 suppl 7):6–16.
24. Nachemson AL. Disc pressure measurements. Spine 1981;6:93.
25. Snook SH, Webster BS, McGorry RW, et al. The reduction of chronic nonspecific low back pain through the control of early morning lumbar flexion: a randomized controlled trial. Spine 1998;23:2601–7.
26. Donelson R, Silva G, Murphy K. The centralization phenomenon: its usefulness in evaluating and treating referred pain. Spine 1990;15:211.
27. Adams MA, May S, Freeman BJ, et al. Effects of backward bending on lumbar intervertebral discs. Relevance to Phys Ther treatments for low back pain. Spine 2000;25(4):431–7.
28. Ingber R. Iliopsoas myofascial dysfunction: a treatable cause of "failed" low back pain syndrome. Arch Phys Med Rehabil 1989;70:382–6.
29. Feibert I, Keller CD. Are "passive" extension exercises really passive? J Orthop Sports Phys Ther 1994;19(2):111–6.
30. Cherkin DC, Deyo RA, Battie M, et al. A critical evaluation of the methodology of a low-back pain clinical trial. A comparison of physical therapy, chiropractic manipulation, and provision of an educational booklet for the treatment of patients with low back pain. N Engl J Med 1998;339:1021–9.
31. Johannsen F, Remvig L, Kryger P, et al. Exercises for chronic low back pain: a clinical trial. J Orthop Sports Phys Ther 1995;22(2):52–9.
32. Mellin G. Physical therapy for chronic low back pain: correlation between spinal mobility and treatment outcome. Scand J Rehabil Med 1985;17:163–6.

33. Kisner C, Colby LA. The spine: traction procedures. In: Therapeutic exercise: foundations and techniques. 3rd edition. Philadelphia: FA Davis Co; 1996. p. 575–91.

34. Graham N, Gross A, Goldsmith C. Mechanical traction for mechanical neck disorders. A systematic review. J Rehabil Med 2006;38:145–52.

35. Van der Heijden GJ, Beurskens AJ, Koes BW, et al. The efficacy of traction for back and neck pain: a systematic, blinded review of randomized clinical trial methods. Physical Therapy 1995;75:93–104.

36. Hurwitz E, Moregenstern H, Harber P, et al. A randomized trial of chiropractic manipulation and mobilization for patients with neck pain: Clinical outcomes from the UCLA neck pain study. Am J Public Health 2002;92(10):1634–41.

37. Butler DS. Mobilisation of the nervous system. Edinburgh: Churchill Livingstone; 1991.

38. Kolber M, Beekhuizen K. Lumbar stabilization: an evidence-based approach for the athlete with low back pain. J Strength Cond Res 2007;29(2):26–37.

39. Press J. Core strength and the overhead athlete: does core training work. Presented at: Injury Prevention and Treatment Techniques: Baseball Medicine Conference. Washington, DC Jan 9, 2009.

40. Moseley GL, Hodges PW, Gandevia SC. Deep and superficial fibers of lumbar multifidus are differentially active during voluntary arm movements. Spine 2002; 27(2):E29–36.

41. Watkins. Available at: http://watkinsspine.com. Accessed May 12, 2009.

Rehabilitation of Ankle and Foot Injuries in Athletes

Lisa Chinn, MS, ATC, Jay Hertel, PhD, ATC*

KEYWORDS

- Achilles Tendinosis • Ankle sprain • Plantar fasciitis
- Therapeutic exercise • Turf toe

The foot and ankle are among the most common sites for acute and chronic injuries in athletes and other physically active individuals.[1] Although seldom life threatening, they often have detrimental effects on sport activity and participation. When an injury to the foot or ankle occurs, athletes are limited in their abilities to run, jump, kick, and change directions. Thus, the treatment and rehabilitation of these injuries are crucial in returning athletes to full participation at full function. When managing injuries of the foot and ankle, all of the typical clinical considerations must be thought of (type of injury, severity, healing time, type and level of activity, and so forth), but it is also important to consider other factors, such as foot type; biomechanics; footwear worn during activity; and external supports, such as bracing or taping. The foot is the base of the lower-quarter kinetic chain, thus, if rehabilitation and treatment is not managed properly, an injury to the foot or ankle can ultimately cause secondary injuries elsewhere up the chain.

BIOMECHANICS OF NORMAL WALKING

For all sports medicine specialists, evaluation of gait is important for the rehabilitation of lower-extremity injuries. Understanding the normal gait pattern will enable a clinician to identify and correct improper compensations after injury. The identification of gait abnormalities should play a key component in deciding to refer patients for supervised rehabilitation. The movement of the lower extremity during normal walking and running can be divided into two phases: the stance phase and the swing phase.

The stance, or support, phase starts with initial contact at heel strike and ends at toe-off. This phase has two important functions. First, at heel strike, the foot acts like a shock absorber to the impact forces and then the foot adapts to the surface. Secondly, at toe-off the foot functions as a rigid level to transmit the force from the foot to the surface. At initial contact, the subtalar joint is supinated and there is an

University of Virginia, Kinesiology Program, Exercise and Sport Injury Laboratory, 210 Emmet Street South, Charlottesville, VA 22904-4407, USA
* Corresponding author.
E-mail address: jhertel@virginia.edu (J. Hertel).

Clin Sports Med 29 (2010) 157–167
doi:10.1016/j.csm.2009.09.006
0278-5919/09/$ – see front matter © 2010 Elsevier Inc. All rights reserved.

external rotation of the tibia. As the foot loads, the subtalar joint moves into a pronated position until the forefoot is in contact with the ground. The change in subtalar motion occurs between initial heel strike and 20% into the support phase of running. As pronation occurs at the subtalar joint the tibia will rotate internally. Transverse plane rotation occurs at the knee joint because of this tibial rotation. Pronation of the foot unlocks the midtarsal joint and allows the foot to assist in shock absorption and to adapt to the uneven surfaces. It is important during initial impact to reduce the ground reaction forces and to distribute the load evenly on many different anatomical structures throughout the foot and leg. Pronation is normal and allows for this distribution of forces on as many structures as possible to avoid excessive loading on just a few structures. The subtalar joint remains in a pronated position until 55% to 85% of the support phase, when maximum pronation is concurrent with the body's center of gravity passing over the base of support. From 70% to 90% of the support phase, the foot begins to resupinate and will approach the neutral subtalar position. In supination, the midtarsal joints are locked and the foot becomes stable and rigid to prepare for push off. This rigid position allows the foot to exert a greater amount of force from the lower extremity to the surface. The swing phase begins immediately after toe-off and ends just prior to heel strike. During the swing phase the leg is moved from behind the body to a position in front of the body.[2]

LATERAL ANKLE SPRAIN

Lateral ankle sprains are common acute injuries suffered by athletes.[1,3] The most common mechanism for a lateral ankle sprain is excessive inversion and plantar flexion of the reafoot on the tibia. The injured ligaments are located on the lateral aspect of the ankle and include the anterior talofibular, the posterior talofibular, and the calcaneofibular.[4]

With lateral ankle sprains, the severity of the ligament damage will determine the classification and course of treatment. In a grade 1 sprain, there is stretching of the ligaments with little or no joint instability. Pain and swelling for a grade 1 sprain are often mild and seldom debilitating. After initial management for pain and swelling of the grade 1 sprain, rehabilitation can often be started immediately. Time loss from physical activity for a grade 1 sprain is typically less than 1 week. Grade 2 sprains occur with some tearing of ligamentous fibers and moderate instability of the joint. Pain and swelling are moderate to severe and often immobilization is required for several days. With a grade 3 sprain, there is total rupture of the ligament with gross instability of the joint. Pain and swelling is so debilitating that weight bearing is impossible for up to several weeks.[5]

Rehabilitation Expectations

With lateral ankle sprains, regaining full range of motion, strength, and neuromuscular coordination are paramount during rehabilitation. Isometrics and open-chain range of motion can be completed by those patients who are non-weight bearing. Range of motion should focus on dorsiflexion and plantar flexion and be performed passively and actively as tolerated. During early rehabilitation, towel stretches, and wobble board range of motion should be introduced as tolerated. Stationary biking can aid dorsiflexion and plantar flexion motion in a controlled environment while also providing a cardiovascular workout for the athlete. Clinicians can also incorporate joint mobilizations to aid in dorsiflexion range of motion.[6] Hydrotherapy is an excellent means to work on range of motion while also gaining the benefits of hydrostatic pressure.

Once weight bearing is tolerated, middle-stage rehabilitation is started. This stage includes balance and neuromuscular control exercises and continued range of motion exercises as tolerated. Balance activities should progress from double-limbed stance to single-limb stance and from a firm surface to progressively more unstable surfaces (**Fig. 1**). Closing the eyes or incorporating perturbations can further challenge patients. Patients can be asked to throw and catch weighted balls, perform single-leg squats, and perform single-limb balance and reaching exercises.[7] Regaining and maintaining range of motion should be continued. Wobble board training and slant board stretches are also important to focus on heel cord stretching.

Increased strengthening exercises should be started once swelling and pain is controlled. Initially, dorsiflexion and plantar flexion strength should be focused on. Weight-bearing calf raises and squats are examples of excellent beginning exercises. As the ligaments heal, inversion and eversion strengthening should be added as tolerated. Resistance bands and ankle weights are a good means to gain strength in all planes of motion (**Fig. 2**). Clinicians can integrate diagonal exercises (ie, combined plantar flexion/inversion and dorsiflexion/eversion) to isolate motions at the talocrural joint.

During this time, it is paramount for clinicians to re-educate athletes on the proper mechanics of walking. Once range of motion and strength is regained, functional activities are included. Functional rehabilitation exercises should begin with simple, uniplanar exercises, such as walking and jogging in a straight line. Once the athlete can perform these without a pain or a limp, hops, jumps, skips, and change of direction can be added. Have the athlete perform 10 jumps for distance on the uninvolved limb and challenge them to match the distance with the involved limb. Do the same for

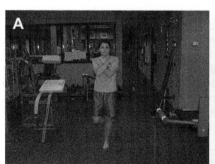
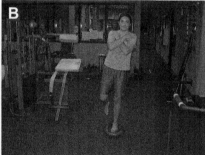
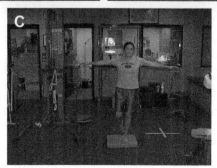

Fig. 1. Balance training exercises include single-limb standing. These exercises can be progressed by changing arm position, closing the eyes, and adding an unstable surface under the foot (*A, B, C*).

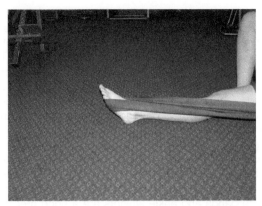

Fig. 2. Strength training may be performed with resistance tubing exercises.

jumps for height. As cutting is started, begin with wide-arching turns and progress to tighter, sharper, and faster cuts. Athletes should be challenged to perform lateral movements as well such as shuffling and carioca. As patients become more comfortable and functional, have them perform rehabilitation wearing the typical shoe/cleat for the sport and progress to more sport-specific activities.

Depending on the severity of the ankle sprain, fear avoidance may cause the athlete to alter play and be at a higher risk for re-injury or injury to another location. Also, some sport-specific skills may need to be reconditioned. Participation in the sport should start with non-contact drills and progress to contact drills and finally to full scrimmage.

Criteria for Full Competition

Full return to activity should be a gradual progression to stress the ligaments without causing further harm. Full activity should be allowed once the athlete has complete range of motion, 80% to 90% of pre-injury strength, and a normal gait pattern including the ability to perform sport-specific tasks, such as cutting and landing without compensation because of the injury. The athlete should be capable, without pain or swelling, to complete a full practice.

Clinical Pearls

- Challenge patients with home exercises. Have patients try to balance on involved limb while brushing teeth and progress to eyes shut while brushing their teeth and balancing.
- Have rehabilitation clinicians perform talocrural and tibiofibular joint mobilizations to increase dorsiflexion.
- Perform exercises with shoes on and off to alter the planter cutaneous feedback.
- Using a 10 to 20 yard area, have patients walk on toes back and forth. Repeat walking with toes pointed in, toes pointed out, and on heels (toes in the air).
- Ask patients to perform 10 single-leg jumps in a row on the involved limb as high as possible, while watching their face. If patients can complete without grimacing, it is safe to start functional rehabilitation.

Patient Education

The leading predisposing factor for an ankle sprain is a history of an ankle sprain.[8] An estimated 30% of all individuals who suffer an initial ankle sprain will develop chronic ankle instability.[4] Thus, patients need to know that inadequate treatment and rehabilitation of an ankle sprain has a great likelihood of leading to future problems.

Patients, coaches, and parents often have the mindset that a lateral ankle sprain is not serious and players can return quickly. However, in many cases health care services are not sought by individuals suffering an ankle sprain.[9] It is critical for all stakeholders to understand the high frequency of residual symptoms and recurrent sprains.[10] The importance of allowing the ligaments to heal, regaining full range of motion, strength, and balance prior to returning to activity must be emphasized to patients. If, while doing rehabilitation, swelling returns, patients must know that they did too much.

Prophylactic Support

Prophylactic support is often used after an ankle sprain to provide mechanical stability. Depending upon individual preference and budget, athletes can use tape or a variety of braces (lace-up, stirrup), or an elastic-type configuration. Taping and bracing reduce the risk of recurrent ankle sprains in athletes.[11] Advantages of braces include ease of application and cost effectiveness. Braces also provide the athlete with proprioceptive stimulation, which implies an improve proprioception and sensory feedback.[12] Taping, on the other hand, can be custom designed for the specific athlete, sport, and instabilities.

OTHER ANKLE SPRAINS

Although less common, medial and syndesmotic ankle sprains often result in more severe injuries causing longer time to heal and rehabilitate. Medial ankle sprains occur with a mechanism of excessive eversion and dorsiflexion, causing the deltoid ligament to be injured. Patients who have medial ankle sprains will often present with swelling and discoloration on the medial aspect of the ankle and unwillingness to bear weight.

Syndesmotic sprains occur with disruption of the interosseous (or syndesmotic) ligament that stabilizes the inferior tibiofibular joint. Injury to this ligament occurs with excessive external rotational or forced dorsiflexion. Syndesmotic sprains may occur in isolation or in combination with medial or lateral ankle sprains. Because of limited blood supply and difficulty in allowing the injured ligament to heal unless the ankle is immobilized, injuries to the syndesmotic ligaments often take months to heal.[13] Patients who have syndesmotic sprains often present with a lack of swelling, but will be extremely tender over anterior aspect of the distal tibiofibular joint.

Rehabilitation Expectations

Initial treatment for medial and syndesmotic sprains is often immobilization and crutches. During this time, swelling and pain management are the primary concerns. The length of time of immobilization will vary among patients and will depend on the severity of the sprain. While immobilized, patients can work on controlled open-chain range of motion, focusing on dorsiflexion and plantar flexion. During this time, inversion and eversion should be held to a minimum. During early rehabilitation, nothing should increase pain or swelling to the area.

Once weight bearing is tolerated, crutches should be used at a minimum. Gait training may be needed to ensure patients are not compensating in any way, which may cause secondary injury. At this point, rehabilitation will follow the progression as stated earlier in the lateral ankle section. Rehabilitation concerns include: pain and swelling, range of motion, strength, balance and neuromuscular control, and functional exercises.

Criteria for Full Competition

Full return to activity should be a gradual progression to stress the ligaments without causing further harm. Full activity should be allowed once the athlete has complete range of motion, 80% to 90% of pre-injury strength, and the ability to perform gait activities (eg, running and changing direction) without difficulty. The athlete should be capable, without pain or swelling, to complete a full practice.

Patient Education

With medial and syndesmotic sprains, patience is the most important thing for patients to learn. The healing of the medial and syndesmotic ligaments takes time, sometimes up to several months, to fully heal. The difference in the expectations of these injuries compared with lateral ankle sprains must be emphasized to all stakeholders so that realistic expectations for return to play can be understood.

PLANTAR FASCIITIS

Plantar fasciitis is the catchall term that is commonly used to describe pain on the plantar aspect of the proximal arch and heel. The plantar fascia is an aponeurosis that runs the length of the sole of the foot and is a broad, dense band of connective tissue. It is attached proximally to the medial surface of the calcaneus and fans out distally, attaching to the metatarsophalangeal articulations and merges into the capsular ligaments. The plantar aponeurosis assists in maintaining the stability of the foot and secures or braces the longitudinal arch.

Plantar fasciitis is caused by a straining of the fascia near its origin. The plantar fascia is under tension with toe extension and depression of the longitudinal arch. During normal standing (weight bearing principally on the heel), the fascia is under minimal stress, however, when the weight is shifted to the balls of the feet (running) the fascia is put under stress and strain. Often, planar fasciitis is a result of chronic running with poor technique; poor footwear; or lordosis, a condition in which the increased forward tilt of the pelvis produces an unfavorable angle of foot strike when there is considerable force exerted on the ball of the foot.[14]

Patients who are more prone to plantar fasciitis include: those with a pes cavus foot; excessive pronation; overweight; walking, running, or standing for long periods of time, especially on hard surfaces; old, worn shoes (insufficient arch support); and tight Achilles tendon.[14] Patients will present with pain in the anterior medial heel, usually at the attachment of the plantar fascia to the calcaneus. The pain is particularly noticeable during the first couple of steps in the morning or after sitting for a long time. Often the pain will lessen as patients move more, however, the pain will increase if patients are on their feet excessively or on their toes often. Upon inspection, the plantar fascia may or may not be swollen with crepitus. Patients' pain will increase with forefoot and toe dorsiflexion.

Rehabilitation Expectations

Depending on patients' compliance, plantar fasciitis can be a very treatable minor injury with symptoms lasting days. However, without proper treatment and patients' compliance, plantar fasciitis can linger for months or even years.

Initial treatment of plantar fasciitis starts with pain control. Rest is extremely important at this time; patients should not begin performing any unnecessary weight bearing activities. Patients should also be wearing comfortable, supportive shoes when walking is necessary. Adding a heel cup or custom foot orthosis to patients' shoes may relieve some of the pain at the plantar fascia insertion.[15] During this time, regaining full dorsiflexion range of motion of the foot and of the big toe is vital. Towel stretches, slant board stretches, and joint mobilizations administered by a rehabilitation clinician will aid in the return of dorsiflexion range of motion.

After pain is reduced, strengthening exercises can be incorporated into rehabilitation. The focus should be in strengthening the smaller extrinsic and intrinsic muscles of the foot. Towel crutches, big toe-little toes raises, and short-foot exercises[16] are good examples of strengthening exercises (**Fig. 3**). Throughout the treatment and rehabilitation process, soft-tissue work, such as cross-friction massage, may aid in the alleviation of symptoms.

Criteria for Full Competition

Although athletes can often continue to participate fully while suffering from plantar fasciitis, it should be understood that the longer activity is continued, the longer the symptoms will linger. For best recovery of this injury, extra activity should not be started until the athlete is able to walk a full day without any pain. Once daily activities are tolerated, activity can slowly be increased until full participation is reached. Throughout the rehabilitation and participation progression, stretching should occur often throughout the day.

Clinical Pearls

- While sitting, roll on a ball (tennis ball, golf ball, and so forth) underneath the medial longitudinal to stretch the plantar fascia.
- Fill a paper cup with water and freeze it; roll on the frozen cup to get the benefits of cold while also stretching the plantar fascia.
- Before getting out of bed in the morning, put on shoes with good arch support to provide the plantar fascia support upon weight bearing.
- Sleep with feet off the end of the bed to allow some dorsiflexion while sleeping.
- Wear a night splint that will keep foot in a dorsiflexed or neutral position.
- Stretching often throughout the day for a short period of time is more beneficial then stretching once a day for a long period of time.
- Do not wear high heels or other shoes with no support (eg, sandals) during the day.

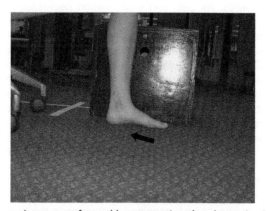

Fig. 3. Short foot exercises are performed by contracting the plantar intrinsic muscles in an effort to pull the metatarsal heads towards the calcaneus. Emphasis should be placed on minimizing extrinsic-muscle activity.

Patient Education

Plantar fascia tends to be a cyclical injury. Athletes will repetitively suffer from this injury because after the initial injury, the cause of the injury is not treated, only the symptoms. Patients who have plantar fasciitis need to have their gait biomechanics thoroughly evaluated, and if necessary, be fitted for custom orthotics.[15]

ACHILLES TENDONITIS

Achilles tendonitis is an inflammatory condition that involves the Achilles tendon or its tendon sheath. Achilles tendonitis is the most common overuse injury reported in distance runners.[17] Although Achilles tendonitis is generally a chronic condition, acute injury may also occur. Typically, athletes will suffer from gradual pain and stiffness about the Achilles tendon region, 2 to 6 cm proximal to the calcaneal insertion. The pain will increase after running hills, stairs, or an increased amount of sprints (running on toes). Upon evaluation, the gastrocnemius and soleus muscle testing may be normal, however, flexibility will be reduced. Having patients perform toe raises to fatigue will show a deficit compared with the uninvolved limb. Inspection of the area may feel warm to the touch and pain, tenderness, and crepitus may be felt with palpation. The tendon may appear thickened, indicating a chronic condition.

Rehabilitation Expectations

Healing of Achilles tendonitis is a slow process because of the lack of vascularity to the tendon. Initially, patients will feel comfortable by placing less stress to the area by wearing a heel cup. Resting and activity modification is important during the initial healing stages. The clinician needs to emphasize the importance of allowing the tendon to heal. During this time, cross-friction massage can be started to the area to break down adhesions and promote blood flow to the area.

Stretching and strengthening of the gastrocnemius-soleus complex should be incorporated as tolerated by patients. Towel stretching and slant board stretching should be done throughout the day. As range of motion is restored, the heel cup should be removed to reduce the chances of adaptive shortening of the muscles and tendon. Progressive strengthening, including toe raises and resistive tubing, should be incorporated at the beginning of rehabilitation. Sets should start low with low repetitions and gradually increase to low sets with high repetitions for endurance as tolerated by patients. As pain and inflammation decreases, machine weights, lunges, and sport-specific exercises can be added. Eccentric exercises for the triceps surae often have beneficial results in patients with Achilles tendonitis.[18]

Patients' foot structure and gait mechanics should be evaluated for possible orthotic benefits. Often Achilles tendonitis is a result of overpronation, an abnormality that can be addressed with foot orthoses.[19] When range of motion, strength, and endurance has returned, athletes should slowly progress into a walking and jogging program. Workouts should be done on a flat surface when possible. The walking and jogging program should start out with slow mini-bursts of speed. The program is to increase the amount of stress the Achilles tendon can tolerate; it is not to improve overall endurance. Running and sprinting can be increased, as tolerated by patients.

Criteria for Full Competition

Athletes should be allowed to compete when full range of motion and strength has returned. The athlete should have regained endurance in the involved limb and be capable of completing a full practice without pain. Depending on the sport, some athletes may be able to compete while suffering from Achilles tendonitis. However, patients should be informed that the condition will not go away without proper rest and treatment.

Patient Education

Patients need to be educated about the risks of Achilles tendonitis, specifically hill running, lack of proper shoes, lack of rest, and flexibility. Hill workouts increase the stress and strain to the gastrocnemius-soleus complex and Achilles tendon. Hill workouts should be done at a maximum of once a week to allow the body time to heal. Similar to any chronic injury to the feet, shoes must be evaluated. Athletes need to learn and understand their foot type and the proper shoes for their foot type. Also, shoes should be replaced every 500 miles or at a maximum of 2 years. Running on old, worn shoes will alter biomechanics and cause stress and strain to the body. Finally, the lack of flexibility is often the main culprit in Achilles tendonitis. The importance of stretching and stretching often should be emphasized.

Prophylactic Support

Initially, heel cups will reduce the tension and stress placed on the Achilles tendon. As flexibility is regained, the heel cup should be gradually reduced to reduce the chances of an adaptive shortening of the tendon. Athletes may also find comfort in a special tape job that will reduce the stress placed on the Achilles tendon.

Patients' foot type and gait mechanics should be evaluated for possible use of custom orthotics. Achilles tendonitis can often be attributed to over pronation during gait. A custom orthotic will be able to adjust athletes' gait to reduce this abnormality.

TURF TOE

Tuft toe is a hyperextension injury of the great toe, causing a sprain to the metatarsophalangeal joint and damage to the joint capsule. Turf toe can be either an acute or a chronic condition. An acute turf toe often occurs when athletes' shoes stick into the ground while they are trying to stop quickly. The shoe sticks as the patients' body weight shifts forward, causing the big toe to jam into the shoe and ground. The chronic condition occurs from frequent running or jumping in shoes that allow excessive great-toe motion. This mechanism of injury may occur on natural or synthetic surfaces.[20]

Athletes who have turf toe will present with pain at the first metatarsophalangeal joint. Swelling and stiffness may be present; however, pain, especially with great-toe extension, is the primary symptom. Rehabilitation of turf toe typically requires several weeks. If left untreated, turf toe can lead to permanent decrease in range of motion and osteoarthritis arthritis.[20]

Rehabilitation Concerns

Patients suffering from turf toe respond best with rest and an adjustment made to their shoes. Pain management should be of primary concern to the clinician. When pain and swelling have been reduced, the athlete should start performing toe extension and flexion exercises, such as toe crunches and short-foot exercises. Joint mobilizations should be added to the treatment protocol to aid in pain and increase range of motion. When pain and swelling is reduced, the athlete may begin to progress into athletic activities. Protecting the great toe with a stiff forefoot insert or great-toe taping may increase athletes' comfort.

Criteria for Full Competition

Athletes are able to return to full competition when any pain and swelling has resolved. Toe taping and shoe inserts often allow athletes who have turf toe to continue practicing and participating while suffering from this injury.

Pearls of Wisdom

- Have patients wear stiff insoled shoes to prevent excessive motion.
- Great-toe joint mobilizations can be incorporated to reduce pain and increase motion.

Patient Education

Patients should be aware that if left untreated, turf toe may cause permanent decreased range of motion in the great toe and bone spurs may develop. Although athletes can often play with turf toe, rest and pain management is the most beneficial for athletes. Without prevention of excessive extension of the great toe, symptoms of turf toe may disappear with rest just to return when the athlete returns to activity.

Prophylactic Support

Athletes with turf toe may benefit from adding a steel or other stiff-material insert into the forefoot of the shoes to reduce extension. Taping of the great toe to prevent dorsiflexion may also be done.

SUMMARY

Nearly all lower-extremity injuries in athletes will benefit from rehabilitation programs that include therapeutic exercise. Restoring joint range of motion, muscle strength, and neuromuscular coordination should be emphasized as should normal gait mechanics. A graduated return to physical activity that includes sport-specific exercises is recommended, with the primary goal being a safe return to sport while minimizing the risk of recurrent injuries.

ACKNOWLEDGEMENTS

This work was supported by a grant from the National Center for Complementary and Alternative Medicine (1R21AT004195) (PI: J Hertel).

REFERENCES

1. Hootman JM, Dick R, Agel J. Epidemiology of collegiate injuries for 15 sports: summary and recommendations for injury prevention initiatives. J Athl Train 2007;42(2):311–9.
2. Prentice WE. Rehabilitation techniques in sports medicine. 3rd edition. Boston: McGraw-Hill; 1999. p. 513.
3. Fernandez WG, Yard EE, Comstock RD. Epidemiology of lower extremity injuries among U.S. high school athletes. Acad Emerg Med 2007;14(7):641–5.
4. Hertel J. Functional anatomy, pathomechanics, and pathophysiology of lateral ankle instability. J Athl Train 2002;37(4):364–75.
5. Bergfeld J, Cox J, Drez D, et al. Symposium: management of acute ankle sprains. Contemp Orthop 1986;13:83–116.
6. Green T, Refshauge K, Crosbie J, et al. A randomized controlled trial of a passive accessory joint mobilization on acute ankle inversion sprains. Phys Ther 2001; 81(4):984–94.

7. McKeon PO, Ingersoll CD, Kerrigan DC, et al. Balance training improves function and postural control in those with chronic ankle instability. Med Sci Sports Exerc 2008;40(10):1810–9.

8. Beynnon BD, Murphy DF, Alosa DM. Predictive factors for lateral ankle sprains: a literature review. J Athl Train 2002;37(4):376–80.

9. McKay GD, Goldie PA, Payne WR, et al. Ankle injuries in basketball: injury rate and risk factors. Br J Sports Med 2001;35:103–8.

10. Braun BL. Effects of ankle sprain in a general clinic population 6 to 18 months after medical evaluation. Arch Fam Med 1999;8(2):143–8.

11. Olmsted LC, Vela LI, Denegar CR, et al. Prophylactic ankle taping and bracing: a numbers-needed-to-treat and cost-benefit analysis. J Athl Train 2004;39(1): 95–100.

12. Jerosch J, Hoffstetter I, Bork H, et al. The influence of orthoses on the proprioception of the ankle joint. Knee Surg Sports Traumatol Arthrosc 1995;3(1):39–46.

13. Wright RW, Barile RJ, Surprenant DA, et al. Ankle syndesmosis sprains in national hockey league players. Am J Sports Med 2004;32(8):1941–5.

14. Wearing SC, Smeathers JE, Urry SR, et al. The pathomechanics of plantar fasciitis. Sports Med 2006;36(7):585–611.

15. Lee SY, McKeon P, Hertel J. Does the use of orthoses improve self-reported pain and function measures in patients with plantar fasciitis? A meta-analysis. Phys Ther Sport 2009;10(1):12–8.

16. Rothermel SA, Hale SA, Hertel J, et al. Effect of active foot positioning on the outcome of a balance training program. Phys Ther Sport 2004;5(2):98–103.

17. Knobloch K, Yoon U, Vogt PM. Acute and overuse injuries correlated to hours of training in master running athletes. Foot Ankle Int 2008;29(7):671–6.

18. Rees JD, Lichtwark GA, Wolman RL, et al. The mechanism for efficacy of eccentric loading in Achilles tendon injury; an in vivo study in humans. Rheumatology 2008;47(10):1493–7.

19. Donoghue OA, Harrison AJ, Laxton P, et al. Lower limb kinematics of subjects with chronic achilles tendon injury during running. Res Sports Med 2008;16(1): 23–38.

20. McCormick JJ, Anderson RB. The great toe: failed turf toe, chronic turf toe, and complicated sesamoid injuries. Foot Ankle Clin 2009;14(2):135–50.

Return-to-Play Criteria Following Sports Injury

Jim Clover, MED, ATC, PTA*, Jerome Wall, MD, FACS

KEYWORDS

• Competition • Guidelines • Preinjury data • Stakeholders

Returning to competition can be a confusing scenario when all the possible circumstances that might be involved are considered. These circumstances involve an array of individuals, including the athlete, parents, guardians, coaches, family physician, the athletic trainer, and others. The key to a successful outcome is making return-to-play or (RTP) decisions and conveying them in a manner all can understand. It is imperative for the clinician to keep in mind that, when making this decision, his or her primary responsibility is to cause no harm to the athlete, while enabling participation at the highest level possible. The decision will be better understood and accepted if all stakeholders are properly informed.

The criteria for RTP or athletic activity is easy or difficult. In most cases, it is straightforward—an athlete can or cannot physically play. However, in some cases it is confusing. Imagine a male athlete comes to see the clinician with general complaints of a very mild back strain. He walks into the clinic with no problem, jumps up on the table with no pain, and has a clear smile on his face. As the evaluation begins, he says he just came from a physician who told him to stay out of activities for 99 days. The clinician's first thought may be, "Why not 98?" This is an example of how things can be much more distorted and confusing than they should be. The parents then ask for a change in his RTP date because 99 days is too long and too confusing. The clinician has no idea what he or his parents said to the doctor during their previous visit. Then the coach calls the discussion becomes more confusing. The athlete has a mild back strain with no radicular pain, radiographs are negative, and the evaluation results appear benign. How was 99 days chosen as an RTP date? Is there merit in evidence-based practice for such a decision? Further, is this a practical piece of advice that the stakeholders understand? Was there any discussion of a reassessment at any point before the 99-day mark? When designing an RTP criteria, one size does not fit all. However, all programs should be prescribed in a reasonable, clear manner in an effort to provide a safe return to participation.

The SPORT Clinic, 4444 Magnolia Avenue, Riverside, CA 92501, USA
* Corresponding author.
E-mail address: jclover@comgri.com (J. Clover).

Clin Sports Med 29 (2010) 169–175
doi:10.1016/j.csm.2009.09.008   sportsmed.theclinics.com

There are different kinds of RTP programs. Various components comprise the ulti-mate decision. Often, when an athlete is seen in a physician's office or hospital setting, imaging or laboratory results are used as a baseline in assessing return to normal tissue or blood values. Measurements may have been taken at the time of the injury and, in some cases, preinjury data may have been collected. By compar-ison, on-the-field RTP guidelines usually require a different set of decision-making skills. The clinician is not likely to have the luxury of imaging equipment. In most cases, decisions are made more rapidly and in front of an audience. This does not preclude the clinician from performing a thorough history and clinical examination. In fact, it arguably places more weight on such components of the assessment process. In most circumstances, the benefit of a complete medical team is also not available. This leaves those present on the sidelines in a volunteer or other capacity to make the decision. These circumstances can change all the rules for the health care provider as they relate to making sound decisions for an athlete's safe RTP. It is imperative to keep in mind that the absence of resources or personnel does not exempt the medical provider from the consequences of a poor decision or allowing an athlete to take a health risk.[1]

ESTABLISHING GUIDELINES

No single formula can serve as an RTP guideline for all conditions. One procedure that would assist in establishing RTP guidelines would be to set up such guidelines in advance and share them with the coaches, athletes, parents, and all other stake-holders.[2] While specifics may not be included, informing others of who makes the decisions, under what circumstances, and how the safety of the athletes takes priority can alleviate impromptu decisions and unrealistic, unsafe expectations. Confusing or absent criteria and policy can lead to challenges for of the stakeholders. Athletes, parents, and coaches may "doctor shop" until they find the RTP criteria they are look-ing for. This is never a good situation, as it undermines respect for the authority of medical decision making. Pre-established guidelines should include a disclaimer stating who makes the final decision regarding an athlete's RTP. For example, if there is a coach and an athletic trainer, the final decision is made by the athletic trainer. If there is an athletic trainer and physician, then the physician is the responsible party. In most cases where there is an athletic trainer and physician, they work together to make the determination because the athletic trainer is usually with the athlete more and may know the athlete better—particularly from a cognitive and personality perspective. This can have benefits as it relates to understanding the athlete's level-of-pain threshold, normal demeanor, and other intangible personality characteristics. While it is always beneficial to have an ultimate decision maker, collaborative deci-sions that involve all of those who serve as part of the medical team can have advantages.

The outcome of a game—winning or losing—should never have an effect on the RTP decision. There is the story about how Jack Youngblood suffered a fractured left fibula in the 1979 first-round playoffs, then played every defensive down in the title game, Super Bowl XIV. Unfortunately, this has become an RTP standard for some athletes and coaches who feel it is a sign of toughness. This mindset is a major concern for all medical providers because serious symptoms can be overlooked when seen as a sign of weakness. Unfortunately, imitating the performance of those who play through pain or dangerous symptoms, or engage in otherwise risky behaviors, is a sign of toughness and courage to many people in the sporting world.[3] Although, in some cases, playing through discomfort is not additionally harmful, medical providers must focus on deciphering between mere toughness and dangerous signs and symptoms that can lead to further risk of injury with a premature RTP.

ATHLETE'S BEHAVIORAL RESPONSES

As with all people, athletes present different behaviors under different circumstances. These behaviors can be described, though not formally classified, in terms of the athlete's response to injury and reaction to the RTP decision. It is common for an athlete to lose emotional control. These athletes tend to direct much of their emotion toward the injury itself. They may tend to showboat the circumstances in an effort to gauge a reaction from a crowd. It can be very hard to perform an evaluation with constant audience reaction. Pressures of external stimuli can lead to rushed and, oftentimes, poor judgment. Ideally, the athlete is removed from the environment to reduce the risk of an erroneous decision by the medical provider. Even if it is impossible to remove the athlete from the distracting environment and despite the athlete's demeanor, it is still necessary to evaluate seriously the portrayed injury.

Another type of behavior commonly seen is the athlete who sustains an injury and then hides from the medical staff for fear of being taken out of competition. In some cases, the athlete may not act alone. A coach or other players may abet an athlete. In addition, it is common for a parent to keep a child away from the medical staff when caught up in excitement about the game's outcome or their child's playing status. Whatever the cause of initial resistance, once an injured athlete is evaluated the best way to demonstrate that the player is not fit for competition is by using the pertinent procedure set up in RTP guidelines. While no medical provider can be technically at fault for an athlete who does not report symptoms, this does not preclude legal responsibility should an adverse circumstance arise leading to a catastrophic event. Knowing the personalities of individual athletes plays a key role when dealing with those who choose to hide their injuries.

Fortunately, a typical form of behavior following an injury and preparing for an RTP is exhibited by many athletes. These athletes still want to play, but they candidly report pain and abide by the recommendations of the medical staff. These individuals may still challenge the decision; however, though they have a great desire to participate, they fear further damage and risk of injury. These athletes tend comply with suggested treatment interventions and rehabilitation protocols while hoping for an opportunity to return to the game as quickly as possible.

RTP-TESTING PROCEDURES

The basic RTP criteria for musculoskeletal and all other injuries should be shared at the beginning of a season with the coaches, players, administration, and parents. This is establishes the RTP rules and remind the stakeholders that it is the injury that prevents participation, not the medical provider. RTP guidelines should also be shared when an injury occurs.

RTP considerations for musculoskeletal injuries should establish an athlete's available range of motion (active and passive), muscle strength, and functional athletic ability as it relates to the expected standards of play. With lower extremity injuries, for example, many options exist. In some cases, a minor sprain to an ankle can be handled with reinforced adhesive tape, over or under the footwear, providing enough support for the athlete to return safely. Agility testing is often a factor in making such a decision. Tests should be performed to assess the athlete's movement in all directions with full weight bearing. The tests should be conducted so that the athlete is directed to do more than just follow a movement pattern, such as a figure 8 or a 90-degree cut. The tests should incorporate an element of surprise. Testing of sport-specific moves is highly encouraged. These are moves the athlete would have to perform immediately upon RTP under the same pace, resistance, and circumstances. Usually, the athlete is attempting to demonstrate that he or she is ready to participate. Observations by the medical staff should include looking for a limp, grimace, or sign that the athlete is still not fully functional. The medical staff must remove an athlete from play if inability to perform tests results in concern for further injury or damage. A return to activity does not end the responsibility of the medical provider. In fact, it is at this time that an increased attentiveness to the injured athlete is necessary. Close observation of this initial RTP period is necessary to confirm that the decision is correct and that the athlete is safe (**Fig. 1**). Upper extremity injury testing and RTP criteria are similar to that of lower extremity injury: assessment of bilateral strength, range of motion, and other functional movement patterns. In addition to manual muscle-testing procedures, upper extremity strength can be assessed through activities such as push-ups that add additional body weight that a medical provider may not be able to replicate for larger-sized athletes.

With the inclusion of functional movement tests, many of which assess agility, balance, strength, and proprioception, the medical provider can make a close prediction of whether an athlete is physically able to perform in a competitive environment. Not all agility testing results in a clear decision. If doubt exists, it is important to lean toward safety rather than risk. When agility tests are designed correctly, only uninjured athletes will be able to perform them. This will eliminate the need for confrontations with a player or coaches. Although working with athletes in front of an audience may be problematic, testing in the presence of a coach or a parent can be advantageous for the medical professional. Then, all the stakeholders witness the ability or inability of the athlete to perform the task. Granted, there may be some biased perception. However, an athlete clearly unable to perform a test would demonstrate this in the presence of the stakeholders. This would prevent the potential problem of the medical provider conveying the message and being challenged by the athlete's perception of his or her performance and readiness to perform. In some settings, videotaping the

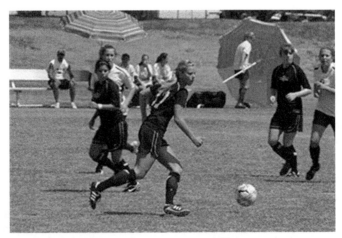

Fig. 1. It is important to watch the athlete once they re-enter for any changes in normal athletic motion.

testing provides objective views and makes clear the medical provider's concern (**Fig. 2**).

In addition to physically assessing an athlete's ability to return to participation, the medical provider must also determine if the athlete has the psychological confidence and readiness to play. If a medical personnel ever suspects that an athlete lacks the mental readiness and confidence to return to play safely, that absence of emotional preparedness should be taken seriously. An athlete who returns to participation lacking mental readiness, especially in a contact or collision sport, may be predisposed for risk of further injury.

Whether RTP decisions are made in an office with much time to ponder the decision in a composed environment or they are made on a field in the heat of a game with the pressures of making a quick decision looming, more should be considered than the athlete's current safety. There are more global or long-term considerations to weigh. What are the long-term versus short-term potential risks involved? What are the known possibilities of increased injury or long-term disability? These, among other questions, need to be answered before an RTP decision is made. Below are examples of additional considerations.

LEVEL OF SPORT
Recreational and Organized Youth Level

In most situations, there will be no medical personnel at practices or games, unless it is a parent of an athlete. It is likely that an medically unqualified coach will make the RTP decisions based solely on their philosophy.

High School Level

There may or may not be an athletic trainer available. The presence of a certified athletic trainer assists tremendously in the RTP decision he or she will probably know the athlete well and objectively and fairly assess readiness to return.

Under unique circumstances, an athlete might try to protect him- or herself if an RTP decision needs to be made and the athlete has already signed for a college scholarship. The athlete's and their parents concern about further injury is complicated by the possibility of losing the scholarship. In other cases, an athlete may be competing for the potential to earn a scholarship, and may want to play despite any risk in order to demonstrate his or her worth in the presence of the scout or coach.

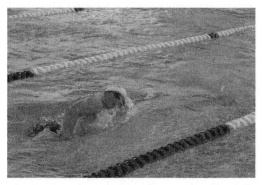

Fig. 2. The eye can only see so much, sometimes the use of a video helps identify problems.

College Level

Most colleges employ one or more certified athletic trainers (based on the total number of athletes participating). In most National Collegiate Athletic Association Division I schools, and in some smaller colleges, the access to medical attention is superior. An athlete with higher level potential might try to protect his or her chances of obtaining a professional contract and a financially lucrative athletic career.

Professional Level

At this level, the athlete plays for a living and is paid for participating. The medical care tends to be superior and accessible, and must meet demands for rapid decisions. This should not result in ill-prepared decisions that can have long-term, adverse outcomes for the athlete and the medical provider. In an effort to protect their livelihood, many professional athletes have health insurance plans (through their teams or as individuals) and long-term disability coverage. Poor RTP decisions that lead to the premature ending of a professional athlete's career can have legal and financial consequences for the medical provider.

INTANGIBLE FACTORS FOR RTP DECISION MAKING

Additional factors come into play for when making an RTP decision for an athlete. These include, but are not limited to

- An athlete's willingness to return. This is a motivational factor that can be influenced by intrinsic and extrinsic factors. This can be assessed through a conversation with the athlete in an effort to gauge their level of interest. Time of the season, number of games remaining, fear of failure, fear of further injury, and closeness of a game or competitive season may all factor into an athlete's willingness to return to participation.
- The parents' willingness to have son or daughter return to participation. Some parents will be forceful in their desire to see their son or daughter play despite the risk of further injury, which may put the athlete in a subservient role to the parent. Conflict with the medical provider can arise. Some parents will take a more conservative approach and, despite limited-to-no further risk of injury, will opt to take no chances regardless of the circumstances.
- Rehabilitation team availability. Depending upon the athlete's access to care, the knowledge to make an RTP decision may or may not be easily available. Access to skilled rehabilitation may also determine the length of time it takes to reach a decision on the safety or risk of participation.
- Insurance coverage. Though insurance or lack thereof should not make a difference in a medical RTP decision, the truth is that can play a role. The type of insurance may determine how soon the athlete has access to medical care and what types of services are provided. In some cases, medical specialty consultations may be influenced. When a rapid decision on the field is not required and one has the time to consider all options in the best interest of an athlete, it is important to know this information.

The bottom line for making decisions about an athlete's RTP status is to do no harm. Whenever possible, allowing an athlete to return to participation should always be considered. Pre-established guidelines on policy and procedure in conveying information to stakeholders can assist during decision-making. While protocols are ever-changing, and new methods often arise regarding evaluation criteria and, in some cases, clearance from injuries (concussion, ligament sprains), it behooves the medical professional to keep abreast of key information related to position statements and decision making in the best interest of the athlete.

ACKNOWLEDGMENTS

The authors wish to thank Chris Gonzales, athletic training graduate student, from California Baptist College on Research.

REFERENCES

1. Clover Jim. Sports medicine essentials: core concepts in athletic training and fitness instruction. 2nd edition. Florence (KY): Cengage Learning; 2007.
2. Rehberg Robb S. Sports emergency care: a team approach. Thorofare (NJ): SLACK; 2005.
3. Michael Sokolove. Warrior girls. New York: Simon & Schuster; 2008.

Strength and Conditioning Techniques in the Rehabilitation of Sports Injury

Greg Werner, MS, MSCC, CSCS, SCCC, ACSM-HFI

KEYWORDS

• Strength • Conditioning • Power • Flexibility
• Sports performance • Coach • Fitness

The role of strength and conditioning coaches is to use current best practices to design exercise programs for athletes to assist them in developing their bodies to resist injury, enhance performance, and compliment the needs of the sport head coach. Additionally, strength and conditioning coaches must develop an open, consistent dialog with the sports medicine staff to aid in the rehabilitation of injured athletes and to collaborate in designing programs to prevent new injures.[1]

As an integral part of an athlete's sports performance team, strength and conditioning coaches are responsible for regular communication with the physicians, physical therapists, athletic trainers, and sport head coach.[1] It is through this constant dialog that strength and conditioning coaches formulate an athlete's training program. If a strength and conditioning coach lacks current information from any member of a sports performance team in regards to an athlete's health status, that program will more than likely be only marginally effective and potentially damaging to the athlete's health and performance. Cross-discipline communication and collaboration are a must for all parties in the sports performance team.

Most often, because of schedule conflicts and logistics, strength and conditioning coaches do not have face-to-face communication with physicians involving an athlete's care. It is a good idea, when applicable, however, that physicians and strength and conditioning coaches meet and exchange dialog pertaining to an athlete's health. In the absence of this communication, the proper channel for this information is for it to be passed down through the performance team via the athletic trainers. Therefore, it is imperative that athletic trainers and strength and conditioning coaches have a daily vehicle of communication regarding athlete health status (ie, face-to-face meeting, daily injury status report, or daily phone call).

Strength and Conditioning Kinesiology, James Madison University, MSC 2301, Box 32 Godwin, Harrisonburg, VA 22807, USA
E-mail address: wernerga@jmu.edu

Clin Sports Med 29 (2010) 177–191
doi:10.1016/j.csm.2009.09.012
0278-5919/09/$ – see front matter © 2010 Elsevier Inc. All rights reserved.

HOW CAN A PHYSICIAN ASSIST THE STRENGTH AND CONDITIONING COACH?

The most important common ground for the performance team members is the athletes whom they serve. With this understanding, strength and conditioning coaches should make a special effort to work up the performance team chain to reach the medical doctors and establish an open relationship of trust and camaraderie. With an open channel of communication between the physician and the strength and conditioning coach, everyone on a sports performance team can have a dialog and a vested interest in athletes' total health status. Conversely, the doors to the weight room and any strength and conditioning venues should be open to any and all members of a sports performance team, and all means of training should be open for discussion between team members. Through mutual respect and open discussion, a sports performance team becomes a better-educated and more stable unit, ultimately leading to a stronger service for athletes' betterment.

STRENGTH AND CONDITIONING PERFORMANCE PRINCIPLES

Scientific research has confirmed that the following principles, when used synergistically, stimulate ability to achieve peak athletic performance.

Progressive Overload

The load or amount of weight lifted for each exercise is the most fundamental component of a strength and power training program.[2,3] The application of load has a crucial impact on the specific development of certain neuromuscular qualities. When muscles are stressed to a level beyond their normal training capacity, overload occurs. This overload causes the active muscles to fatigue to a point of breakdown or catabolism. The body then responds, with the aid of proper nutrition and rest, by building up the affected muscles (anabolism).[4]

It is this building up or anabolic phase that develops new strength, power, size, and endurance within the muscles.[4]

Intensity and volume are the key factors that can be manipulated to progressively control the overload of the neuromuscular system. By increasing the load, intensity is increased, and by increasing repetitions, volume is increased. Each of these methods brings about specific adaptations. Lifting heavy loads for low repetitions develops muscular strength; lifting varied loads explosively develops power; and lifting lighter loads for high repetitions develops muscular endurance.[2,3,5]

Periodization Application

Strength and power eventually plateau and even diminish if the same combinations of sets and repetitions are followed. The way to avoid this is by applying periodization or cycling to training plans. Cycling uses different combinations of volume and intensity, or phases, each translating into different responses by the body. Traditionally, a cycle begins with a base phase and progresses to a strength phase, finishing with a peak phase.[2,3,5]

Split Routine

Whether or not 2, 3, or 4 days per week workout is prescribed, a split routine should be implemented. A split routine means alternating the type of exercises performed or body parts trained on alternate days. An example is performing explosive lifts on Mondays and Thursdays and slower strength lifts on Tuesdays and Fridays. Another example of a split routine is training chest, shoulders, and triceps on Mondays and Thursdays and legs, back, and biceps on Tuesdays and Fridays. The benefits of using a split routine are allowing for greater recovery between workout and greater specialization or specificity.[2,3,5]

Heavy–lighter System

More progress can be made over longer periods of time if maximum loads are not work at during each workout. The heavy–lighter system eliminates overtraining and mental burnout. With it, there is only one maximum workout per week for each type of lifting or body part. The second day is a lighter workout, in which the volume or intensity is reduced. With only one heavy workout a week for the explosive exercises and one for the strength exercises, readiness for physical and mental demands improve. Generally the first workouts of the week are the most challenging days (the body is less fatigued after a weekend of rest), and the last workouts are the lighter.[2,3,5]

Specific Energy System Training

The primary objective of conditioning is to improve the energy capacity of athletes to improve performance. For effective conditioning, training must occur at the same intensity and duration as those at which an athlete competes to develop the proper energy system predominately used (training specificity).

ATP is the immediate energy source for all muscle contractions. It comes from the breakdown of food. It is supplied by the interaction of three types of energy systems. The first system is the ATP-phosphocreatine (PC) system. High-intensity, short-duration activities, such as the 40-yard dash or push press, are performed using energy from this system. Energy is supplied immediately, and the amount of force generated from the muscle contraction is high, but the amount of energy readily available is limited and ATP is depleted within approximately 6 to 10 seconds (**Table 1**).

The second energy system is the lactic acid system (glycolysis). The amount of force generated by this system is less than from the ATP-PC system. This system has two phases. During the first phase, ATP is produced from the breakdown of glycogen in the absence of oxygen and a metabolic by-product called lactic acid is produced. The highest accumulation of lactic acid is reached during activities that last from 1 to 3 minutes. Too much lactic acid builds up when the energy system is depleted. This causes pain, which results in a loss of coordination and force production, as often happens at the end of a 400- or 800-m run.

The third system is the aerobic system. This system is more specific to the slow-twitch muscle fibers used during activities requiring endurance over a long duration at a low intensity. After approximately 3 minutes of low-intensity exercise, ATP is almost completely supplied from the aerobic system.

The system ATP is supplied from depends on the intensity and duration of the exercise. The first step used in setting up a conditioning program is to determine the energy system used by the activity according to the intensity and duration of it.

Table 1
Effect of event duration on primary energy systems used

Duration of Event	Intensity of Event	Primary Energy Systems
0–6 s	Very intense	Phosphagen
6–30 s	Intense	Phosphagen and anaerobic glycolysis
30 s–2 min	Heavy	Anaerobic glycolysis
2–3 min	Moderate	Anaerobic glycolysis and oxidative system
>3 min	Light	Oxidative system

Then a similar type of activity is used for conditioning. That way the proper energy system is trained. Different sports use different energy systems and, therefore, require different metabolic demands (**Table 2**).[2,3,5]

Multiple Joint Actions

In order to optimally develop athleticism, strength and conditioning programs are based on exercises and drills involving multiple joint actions. Sport skills, such as jumping, running, or taking on an opponent, require multiple joint actions timed in the proper neuromuscular recruitment patterns.

An example of this multiple joint action is the execution of the hang clean. It requires joint actions at the hips, knees, ankles, shoulders, elbows, and wrists working together as a unit, generating explosive force. Isolating a single joint action might work for body building to target a single muscle, but athletes need to concentrate on activities involving multiple joint actions to improve functional strength and performance.[2,3,5]

Ground-based Exercises

The majority of sport skills are initiated by applying force with the foot against the ground. When possible, lifting exercises and conditioning drills are selected that apply force with the feet against the ground, such as squats, dead lifts, lunges, hang cleans, push presses, or plyometrics. The more force athletes apply against the ground, the faster they run, the higher they jump, and the more effective they are in sport skills.[2,5]

Table 2
Primary metabolic demands of various sports

Sport	Phosphagen System	Anaerobic Glycolysis	Aerobic Metabolism
Archery	High	Low	—
Baseball	High	Low	—
Basketball	High	Moderate to high	Low
Diving	High	Low	—
Fencing	High	Moderate	—
Field events	High	—	—
Field hockey	High	Moderate	Moderate
Football	High	Moderate	Low
Gymnastics	High	Moderate	—
Ice hockey	High	Moderate	Moderate
Lacrosse	High	Moderate	Moderate
Softball	High	Low	—
Soccer	High	Moderate	High
Swimming, sprint	High	Moderate	—
Swimming, distance	High	Moderate to high	Moderate to high
Tennis	High	Low	—
Track, sprint	High	Moderate to high	—
Track, distance	—	Moderate	High
Volleyball	High	Moderate	—

Explosive Movements

Not only are strength gains determined by the size of the muscles but also many times an athlete gets stronger because of an improved ability of the nervous system to recruit motor units. A motor unit is a motor nerve and all the muscle fibers that it innervates. The more fibers a motor unit consists of, the more force it can generate. Through heavy training ($\geq$80% of maximum) and explosive training, the body learns to recruit more motor units so that more force can be generated.

The amount of force required for a given activity is regulated by the use of two different types of motor units found in the body, fast twitch and slow twitch, which differ in their ability to generate force. The number of fibers a fast-twitch motor unit innervates is greater than that of a slow twitch, and the contractile mechanism of fast-twitch muscle fiber is much larger. These factors combined mean a fast-twitch fiber generates a force 4 times greater than a slow-twitch fiber. Heavy or explosive training allows more fast-twitch muscle fibers to be recruited and in return improves an athlete's performance potential. The aims of anaerobic versus aerobic training differ[2,5] (**Boxes 1** and **2**).

3-D Movement

Sport skills involve movements in the three planes of space simultaneously: forward-backward, up-down, and side-to-side. Strength and conditioning programs improve functional strength and power with exercises and drills approximating these 3-D skills.

In strength and power training, only free weights allow movement in three dimensions simultaneously. This makes the transfer of strength and power easier to merge with the development of sport skills. Machines limit the development of sport skills. For example, when free weights are used, the muscles regulate and coordinate the movement pattern of the resistance, whereas machines use lever arms, guide rods, and pulleys to dictate the path of the movement. An additional benefit of free weights is their ability to help prevent major joint injuries. The smaller synergistic muscle groups involved in free weight exercises develop joint integrity better than machines do due to the balancing action required with free weights. For example, squatting using free weights requires the back and abdominal muscles to stabilize the torso isometrically. This allows the legs and hips to work with the back and abdominals as a unit to perform the lift. In contrast the adjustable seat back on the hip sled or leg press substitutes as the back and abdominal stabilizers restricting movement and isolating muscle contractions to the hips and legs.

When developing a running program, explosive footwork and agility drills similar to specific sport movements are used. It is important for athletes to be quick and to possess breakaway speed, but they must be able to control their bodies and execute change of direction quickly on the field or court to be effective.[2,5]

Box 1
Aims of anaerobic training

To develop speed and power

To develop your anaerobic threshold—the ability to repeatedly perform high-intensity work

To decrease recovery time

Quicker removal of lactate from muscles

Prolong the onset of fatigue

Box 2
Aims of aerobic training

To increase oxygen uptake

To increase the muscle's ability to use oxygen

To increase the body's endurance base

To decrease recovery time

Interval Training

Conditioning programs can be based on interval training principles. Interval training is work or exercise followed by a prescribed rest interval. Programs should be designed to meet the specific conditions of each sport. Interval training stresses not only the work phase but also the recovery phase between work intervals. If a rest period is too short, the amount of energy is not sufficient to meet the demands of the next maximum intensity effort, and force output is reduced. The higher the exercise intensity, the longer the recovery phase should be in relation to work time.[2,5]

STRENGTH AND CONDITIONING TRAINING PHILOSOPHY

Athletics are an integral part of any school's overall educational program, but academics come first. A scholastic or collegiate strength and conditioning program should include these policies:

- Athletes are never asked or expected to participate in a strength and conditioning activity in conflict with their academic obligations.
- The welfare and safety of the athletes is paramount and always takes precedence when they are asked to perform an activity.
- Athletes are never asked or allowed to perform a strength activity that the strength and conditioning staff thinks is beyond their capacity to safely execute.

Athletes competing at a high level are expected to produce performances of elite magnitude to be competitive. In order to prepare athletes to compete at this elite level, training must be intense and physically demanding. The strength and conditioning staff encourage and coach athletes to work at their maximum capabilities and, although all precautions are taken to safeguard against injuries, realistically, injuries are not avoidable.

The strength and conditioning staff are motivators and educators; they lead by guiding rather than ruling. Simple principles that can be adhered to in an effort to guide athletes include

o Athletes need feedback to improve their performance. Strength and conditioning coaches should project positive influence and feedback with the power of attitude and example. They should not berate or denigrate athletes to get a point across. Strength and conditioning coaches should follow a simple, direct approach and concisely and clearly explain the principle-based reasons for everything they do.

o Strength and conditioning coaches should inform athletes as to what is expected of them and reward those who achieve these expectations.

o Strength and conditioning coaches should constantly strive to be creative and innovative in all their endeavors. All staff should be encouraged to bring forth new and better ideas for improving performance, whatever their responsibilities.

o Strength and conditioning coaches should be partners with all those on a sports performance team, working together in the pursuit of the same mission and strategy.[1] They should strongly value team work and want every staff member to be motivated to succeed.

o Strength and conditioning coaches should value integrity. Underscoring all their professional life - their professional image, both on the job and in the community. Every activity must be able to pass the test of public and internal scrutiny at all times. A sports performance program should demand openness and honesty throughout its operations to engender trust and integrity.

A quality strength and conditioning program should be based on the principles of exercise science: kinesiology, exercise physiology and biomechanics, and direct proved experience.[2] Additional considerations include, but are not limited to, the following:

- Do not train athletes to become bodybuilders, power lifters, or Olympics-style weightlifters; rather, train athletes to become better athletes. Train athletes to develop the components of athleticism: strength, power, flexibility, speed, agility, footwork, endurance, metabolic condition, body composition, mental focus, and motivation.
- Utilize the principle of specificity, and, therefore, use free weight training as much as possible. Free weights allow athletes to move athletically and not in a fixed motion pattern, unlike most machines. Train movements and thereby train the muscles that produce these movements, but, realistically, certain movements are not ideally trainable with free weights, in which case, use specific machines.
- Utilize explosive power training (plyometrics, power shrugs, power cleans, push presses, jerks, and power squats). Athletes with great power and explosiveness, for the most part, dominate athletics. If all other factors are equal, an athlete with the greatest power and explosiveness dominates his opponent. Follow a sequential progression to maximize safety and optimize success for all explosive power movements.

DYNAMIC FLEXIBILITY AND MOBILITY

A proper workout should have a prescribed warm-up. A 3-minute total body warm-up (ie, jogging, rope jumping, and total body movement) should always precede a dynamic flexibility series. The warm-up raises the body temperature, increases blood flow to the muscles, and lubricates the joints.[2,6] Always remember warm-up to stretch, do not stretch to warm-up. Dynamic movements are one of the best ways to prepare the body for dynamic workouts. Contrary to old beliefs, the best time to work on static flexibility is at the end of a workout, not in the beginning. After every workout, an athlete should follow a 4- to 6-minute total body static stretching series. An example of a standard dynamic flexibility series is described.[2,6]

Walking High Knees

Purpose: to flex the hips and shoulders and stretch the gluteus, quadriceps, lower back, and shoulders (**Fig. 1**).

Procedure
1. Take an exaggerated high step, driving the knee as high as possible simultaneously pushing up on the toes of the opposite foot.
2. Use the proper arm swing: 90° angle at the elbows, hands swing up to chin level and back beyond rear pocket.

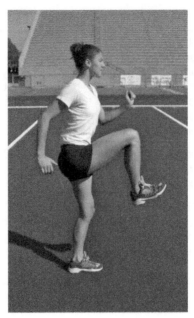

Fig. 1. Walking high knees. (*Photo taken by* Greg Werner. Athlete: Carla Gessler.)

Key point: drive the knees up as high as possible.
Variation: high knees pull; walking high knees as described previously but grab
the knee and pull it up and in with each stride.

Walking Lunge

Purpose: to stretch the gluteus, hamstrings, hip flexors, and calves (**Fig. 2**).

Procedure
1. Step out with a long stride, striking the heel of the forward foot and extending onto
the toes of the back foot.

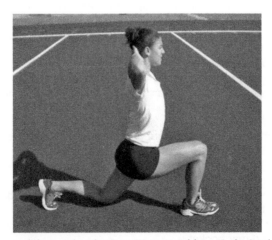

Fig. 2. Walking lunge. (*Photo taken by* Greg Werner. Athlete: Carla Gessler.)

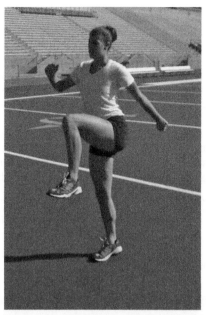

Fig. 3. Walking high knee lunge. (*Photo taken by* Greg Werner. Athlete: Carla Gessler.)

2. Complete the cycle by bringing the trail leg through and standing upright.
    Key points
    1. Position hands behind head while keeping eyes focused forward.
    2. Flex front knee to 90° and keep back knee from striking the ground.

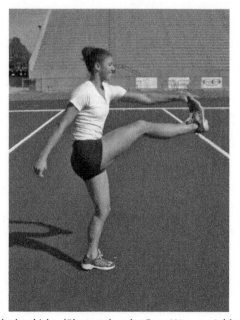

Fig. 4. Walking straight leg kicks. (*Photo taken by* Greg Werner. Athlete: Carla Gessler.)

Walking High Knee Lunge

Purpose: to stretch the gluteus, hamstrings, hip flexors, and calves (**Fig. 3**).

Procedure
1. Drive the forward knee up as high as possible and then step out with a long stride striking the heel of the forward foot and extending onto the toes of the back foot.
2. Complete the cycle by bringing the trail leg through and standing upright.
   Key points
   1. This drill is performed identically to the walking lunge, with the exception of the high knee action.
   2. Position hands behind head with eyes focused forward.
   3. Flex front knee to 90° and keep back knee from striking the ground.

Walking Straight Leg Kicks

Purpose: to stretch the hamstrings, calves, and lower back (**Fig. 4**).

Procedure
1. Walk forward keeping front leg straight.

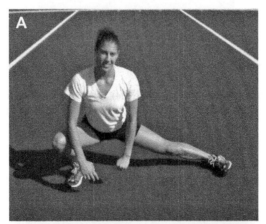

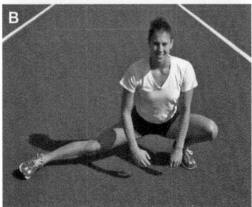

Fig. 5. Walking side lunge, over (*A*) and back (*B*). (*Photo taken by* Greg Werner. Athlete: Carla Gessler.)

2. Kick leg up and touch toes to the fingers of opposite hand.
3. Repeat the cycle with opposite leg.
   Key points
   1. Keep arm extended out parallel with the ground.
   2. On first set of this drill, only kick to 75% capacity; then on second set, kick to full capacity.

Walking Side Lunge, Over and Back

Purpose: to stretch the groin, gluteus, hamstrings, and ankles (**Fig. 5**).

Procedure
1. Keep torso upright and take a long stride out to the side.
2. Lunge out bending forward knee to 90° while keeping trail leg straight.
3. Lower hips and shift body weight to the opposite leg.
4. Recover by bringing the feet together and standing upright.
   Key points
   1. Repeat the drill for 10 yards.
   2. Keep head focused forward with arms hanging down in front of body.

Running Butt Kicks, 20 Repetitions

Purpose: to stretch the quadriceps and hip flexors (**Fig. 6**).

Procedure
1. Begin running by flexing knee and bringing heel back and around to buttocks.
2. Maintain a slight forward lean throughout the drill and stay on the balls of the feet.
3. Complete 20 kicks within 10 yards.

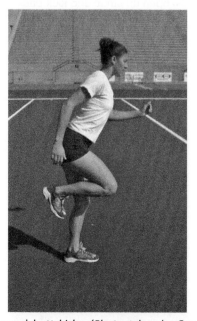

Fig. 6. Running knees forward butt kicks. (*Photo taken by* Greg Werner. Athlete: Carla Gessler.)

Key points
1. Maintain a quick yet shallow arm swing, keep elbows at 90°, and drive hands from chest to front hip pocket.

Running High Knees, 20 Repetitions

Purpose: to stretch the gluteus, quadriceps, low back, and shoulders (**Fig. 7**).

Procedure
1. Execute proper running form; keep elbows at 90° and drive hands up to chin level and back to rear pocket.
2. Stay on the balls of the feet and drive knees up as high as possible, then down as quickly as possible.

Running Carioca

Purpose: to stretch the abductors, adductors, gluteus, ankles, and hips (**Fig. 8**).

Procedure
1. Stay on the balls of the feet with hips in a low semisquat position.
2. Begin the drill by twisting hips and crossing one leg in front of the other, bring trail leg through, and cross lead leg behind the trail leg.
3. Shoulders remain square through the entire drill.

Back Pedal

Purpose: to stretch the hip flexors, quadriceps, and calves.

Procedure
1. Keeping hips and knees bent with shoulders positioned over the balls of the feet.
2. For the first 10 yards, use short choppy steps.
3. For the second 10 yards, open up stride and kick back.

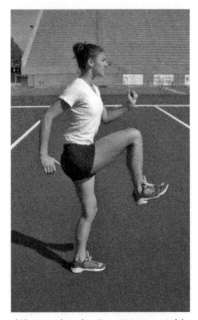

Fig. 7. Running high knees. (*Photo taken by* Greg Werner. Athlete: Carla Gessler.)

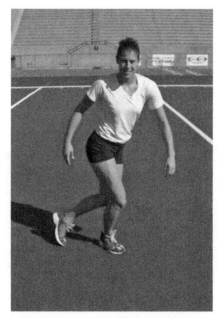

Fig. 8. Running carioca. (*Photo taken by* Greg Werner. Athlete: Carla Gessler.)

Lying Scorpion

Purpose: to stretch the hip flexors, abdominals, quadriceps, and shoulders (**Fig. 9**).

Procedure
1. Lie down in a prone position.
2. While keeping the chest in contact with the ground, cross one leg behind the other to the opposite side of body.

This drill should be done in a continuous manner.

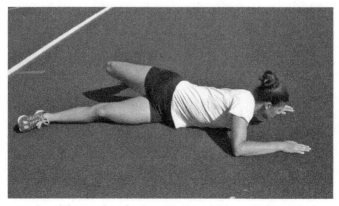

Fig. 9. Lying scorpion. (*Photo taken by* Greg Werner. Athlete: Carla Gessler.)

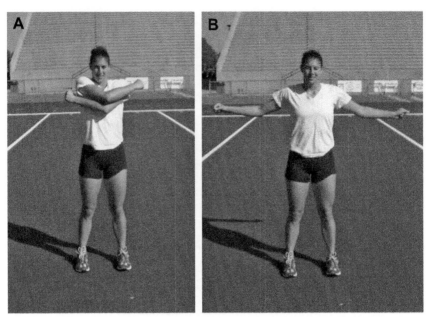

Fig. 10. Arm swings, forward (*A*) and back (*B*). (*Photo taken by* Greg Werner. Athlete: Carla Gessler.)

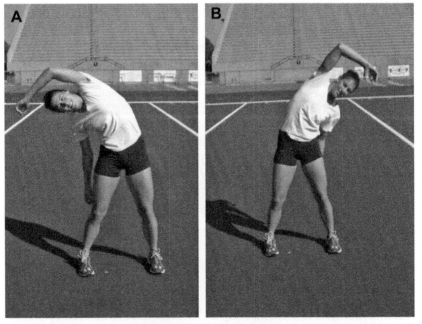

Fig. 11. Side bend, over (*A*) and back (*B*). (*Photo taken by* Greg Werner. Athlete: Carla Gessler.)

Arm Swings, Forward and Back

Purpose: to stretch the chest, shoulders, and upper back (**Fig. 10**).

Procedure
1. Swing arms forward, so they cross, and swing them back as far as possible.
2. This drill should be done in a controlled continuous fashion for 10 repetitions.

Side Bend, Over and Back

Purpose: to stretch the triceps, upper back, abdominals, and obliques (**Fig. 11**).

Procedure
1. Bend to one side while holding opposite arm overhead; quickly reverse direction and stretch the other side.
2. This drill should be done in a controlled continuous fashion for 10 stretches on each side of the body.

Power Skip

Purpose: to further prepare the body for full speed action.

Procedure: the power skip is executed by doing an explosive, exaggerated skip while emphasizing height rather than distance. Emphasize a big arm swing and explosive knee lift.

REFERENCES

1. Werner G. To the weightroom after injury—now. Journal of Pure Power 2002;32–8. Available at: http://www.jopp.us/home.html.
2. NSCA. Essentials of strength training and conditioning. 3rd edition. Human Kinetics: Champaign (IL); 2009.
3. Hatfield, Frederick C. Powerlifting and speed-strength training, 1997.
4. Ivy J, Portman R. Nutrient timing: the future of sports nutrition. North Bergen (NJ): Basic Health Publications; 2004.
5. Epley Boyd. University of Nebraska, Husker power performance principles. Lincoln (NA); 1997.
6. Werner G. Dynamic warm-ups for dynamic performance. Journal of Pure Power 2003;76–81.

Index

Note: Page numbers of article titles are in **boldface** type.

Clin Sports Med 29 (2010) 193–201
doi:10.1016/S0278-5919(09)00087-8
0278-5919/09/$ – see front matter © 2010 Elsevier Inc. All rights reserved.

sportsmed.theclinics.com

Moving?

Make sure your subscription moves with you!

To notify us of your new address, find your **Clinics Account Number** (located on your mailing label above your name), and contact customer service at:

Email: journalscustomerservice-usa@elsevier.com

800-654-2452 (subscribers in the U.S. & Canada)
314-447-8871 (subscribers outside of the U.S. & Canada)

Fax number: 314-447-8029

Elsevier Health Sciences Division
Subscription Customer Service
3251 Riverport Lane
Maryland Heights, MO 63043

*To ensure uninterrupted delivery of your subscription, please notify us at least 4 weeks in advance of move.

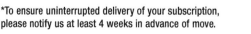

Printed and bound by CPI Group (UK) Ltd, Croydon, CR0 4YY

03/10/2024

01040464-0001